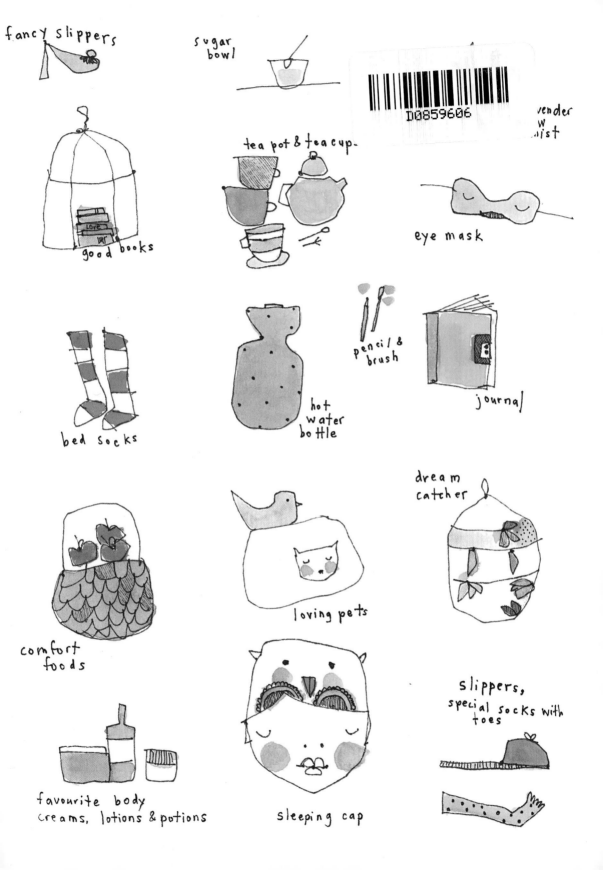

fancy slippers

sugar bowl

tea pot & tea cup

lavender w mist

good books

eye mask

bed socks

hot water bottle

pencil & brush

journal

comfort foods

loving pets

dream catcher

favourite body creams, lotions & potions

sleeping cap

slippers, special socks with toes

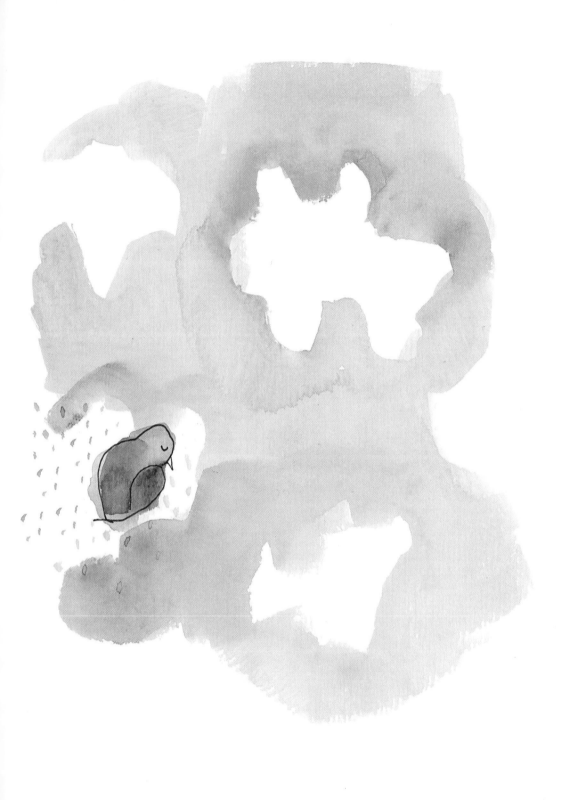

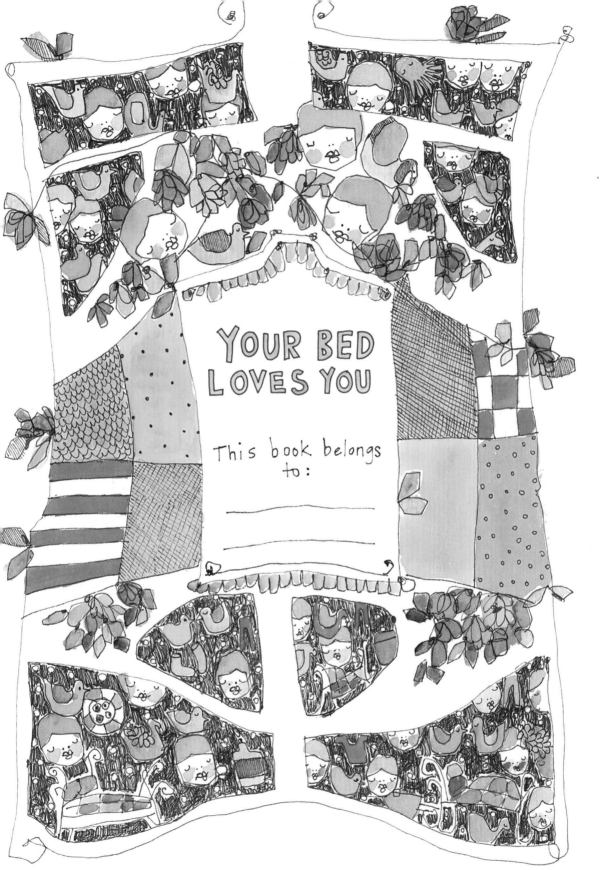

YOUR BED
LOVES YOU

This book belongs
to:

_____

_____

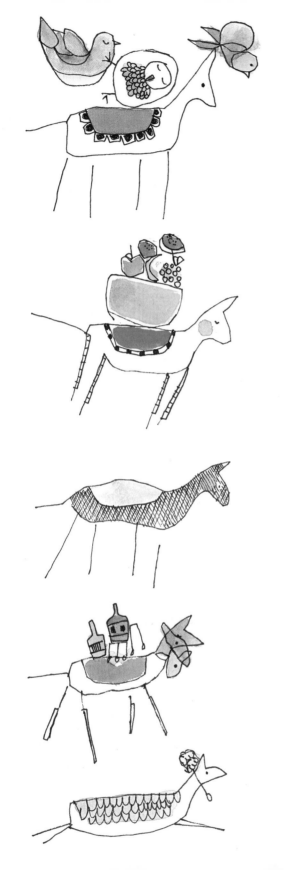

Sleepy ?

Weak ?

Worn out

overwhelmed

just keeping
cosy ?

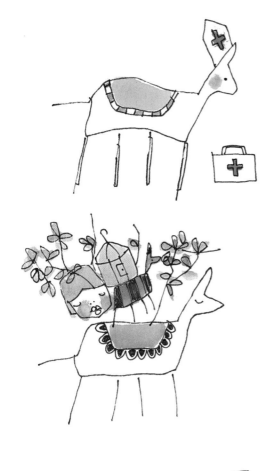

a little bit
unwell ?

a dreamer ?

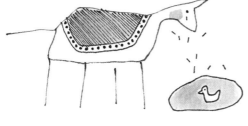

a little bit sad ?

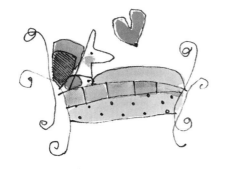

for the love
of bed ? ...

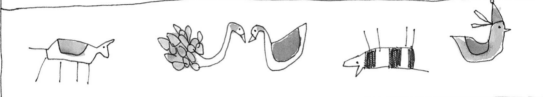

Like all creatures, we human beings have our good and bad times:

Sometimes it is simply so that the best place to be is in bed.

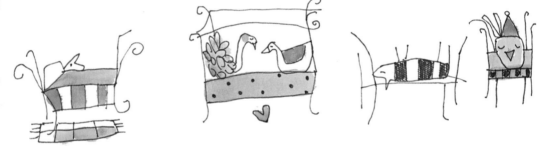

COSY · WARM · HEALING SANCTUARY · QUIET · SECRET · DREAMY · BED.

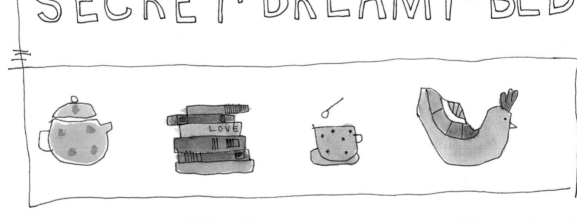

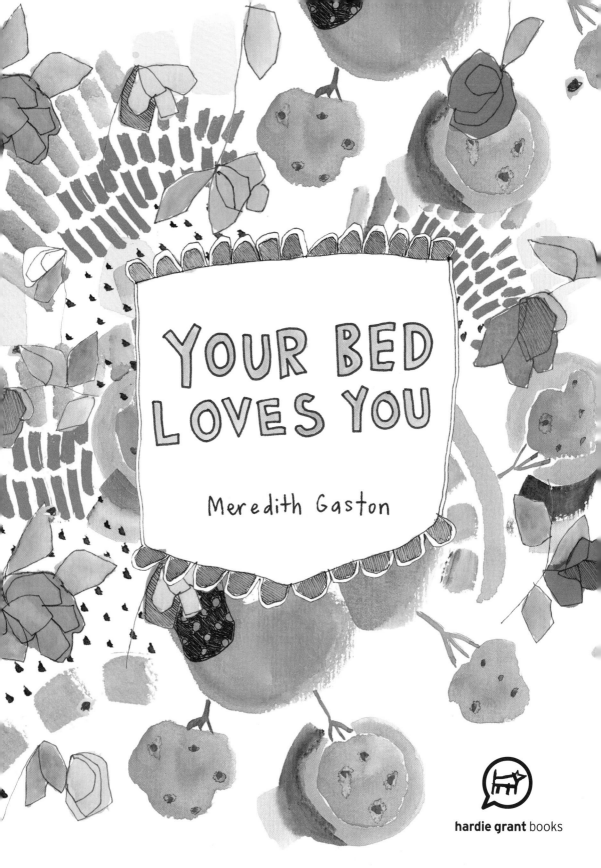

YOUR BED LOVES YOU

Meredith Gaston

hardie grant books

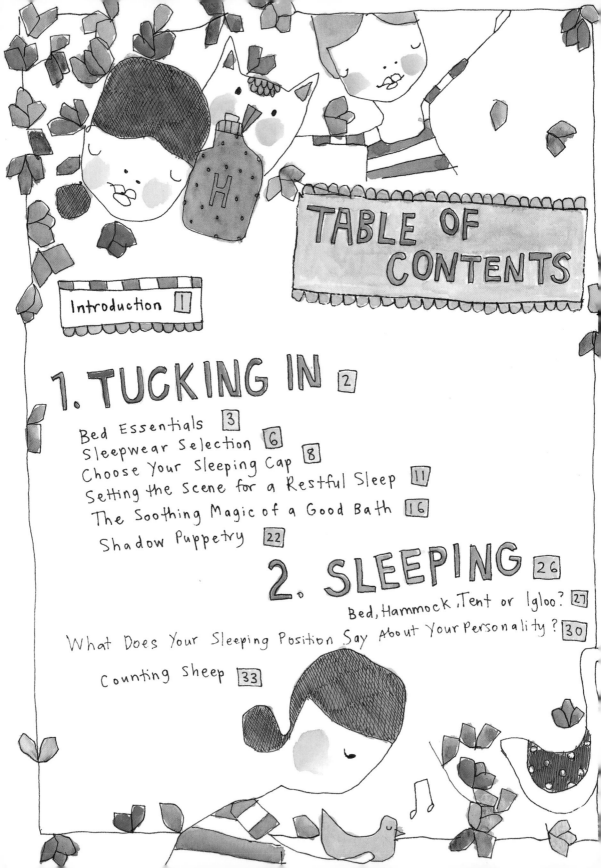

TABLE OF CONTENTS

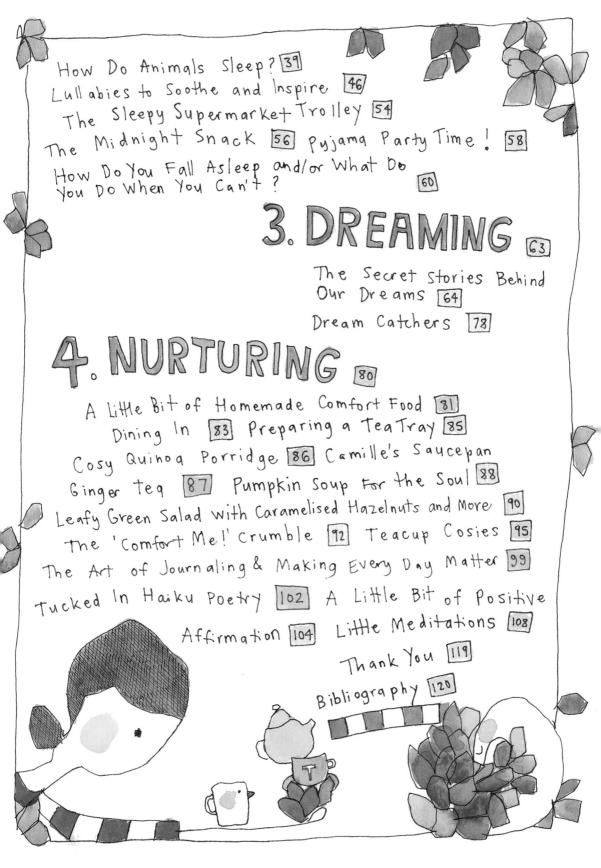

WHETHER YOU ARE YOUNG OR OLD, NIMBLE OR WOBBLY, BED-BOUND ON DOCTOR'S ORDERS OR AT YOUR VERY OWN WHIM, YOUR BED ABSOLUTELY LOVES YOU. EACH CHANCE YOU TAKE TO LET YOUR BED LOVE YOU ACTIVATES YOUR OWN UNIQUE HEALING POWERS, OPTIMISING YOUR COMFORT, VITALITY, MOOD AND MORE.

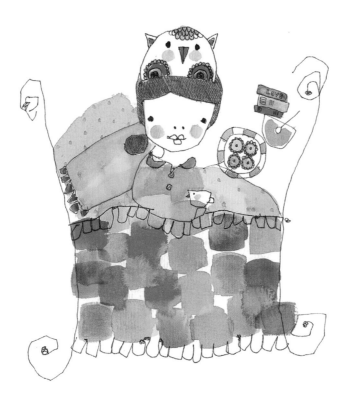

SLEEP POSSESSES VERY SPECIAL HEALING POWERS. As we sleep, our minds and bodies perform various very important functions, recharging us and optimising our wellbeing. Acknowledging how much our beds love us is life-changing, especially in this busy world that values productivity at the expense of quality rest and relaxation.

While some of us may nod off with ease, the idea of sleep may be fraught with worry for others. Wakefulness may make finding slumber challenging, and we might even berate ourselves for our failure to rest and relax. Alas, we needn't become involuntarily nocturnal! There are so many ways to induce restfulness, and to enjoy our beds as a creative, restorative, imaginative and whimsical sanctuaries. Our beds are sacred spaces where we can be ourselves, replenish ourselves, and experience the peace and comfort we deserve.

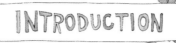

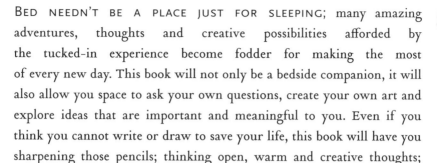

INTRODUCTION

Bed needn't be a place just for sleeping; many amazing adventures, thoughts and creative possibilities afforded by the tucked-in experience become fodder for making the most of every new day. This book will not only be a bedside companion, it will also allow you space to ask your own questions, create your own art and explore ideas that are important and meaningful to you. Even if you think you cannot write or draw to save your life, this book will have you sharpening those pencils; thinking open, warm and creative thoughts; and dusting off that magic treasure chest – your imagination!

We will weave through preparations for tucking in, from organising your bed essentials to setting a tea tray. You might like to choose your own sleeping cap, or consider an appropriate choice of sleepwear for your tucking-in needs.

In the Sleeping section, you'll discover some useful techniques for a restful, replenishing slumber, find out about secret sleep-inducing foods and fragrances, and share in sleeping tips from tucked-in family, friends and strangers from around the world.

If you are curious about the magical meanings behind your dreams or wish to ensure you enjoy good ones, discover the Dreaming pages. You might like to read about dream catchers and borrow some hints to make your own, or decode your sleeping subconscious with an illustrated guide to the most common dream themes and symbols.

Nurturing and being nurtured is so crucial to wellbeing and happiness, so why not treat yourself, treat somebody else or allow yourself to be treated with a hearty, healing pumpkin soup or cup of warm ginger tea? For dessert, why not embrace the power of positive thinking, enjoy a meditation, or make your own personal set of affirmation cards? The wonders of tucked-in creativity are boundless!

So snuggle back, relax, and let yourself be guided through a world of slippers, doonas, dreams, lullabies, tea cups and assorted sleepy facts to get you thinking, dreaming and smiling.

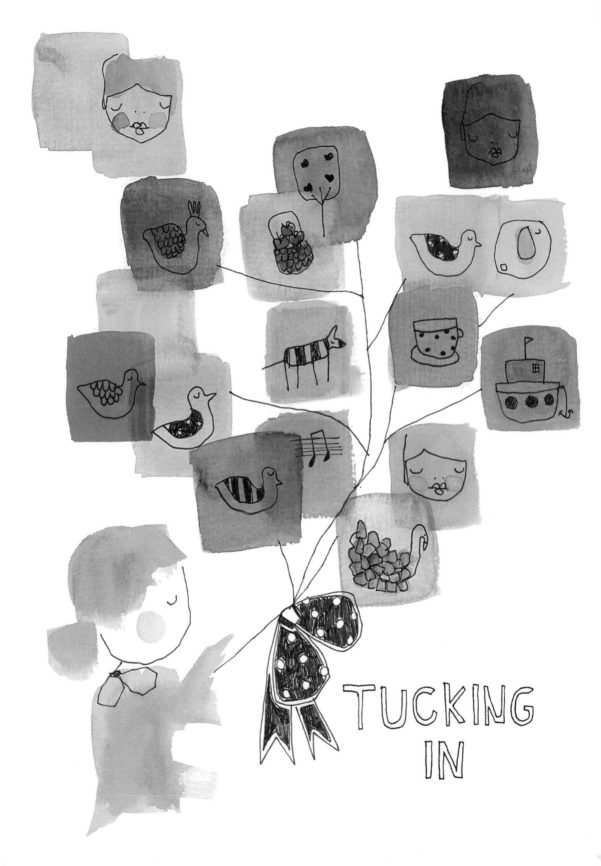

TUCKING
IN

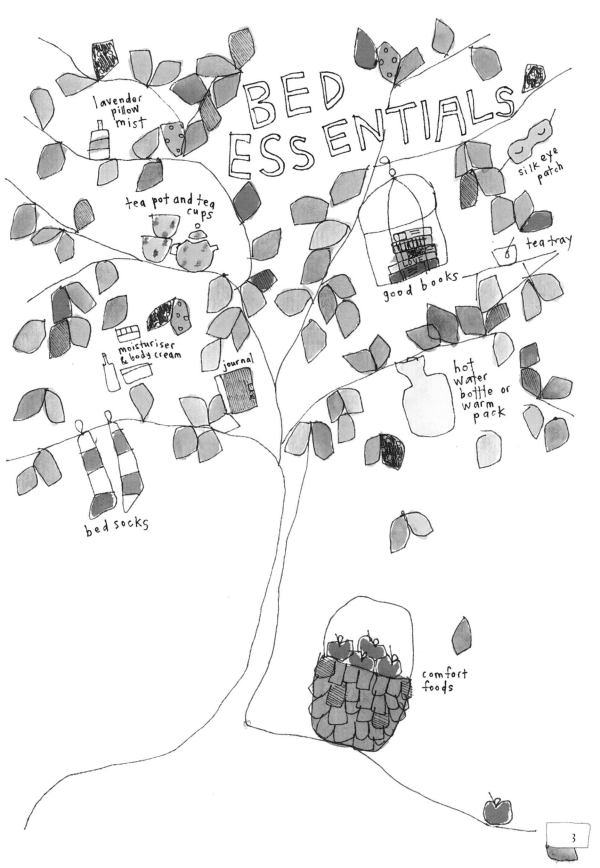

BED ESSENTIALS

lavender pillow mist

silk eye patch

tea pot and tea cups

tea tray

good books

moisturiser & body cream

journal

hot water bottle or warm pack

bed socks

comfort foods

3

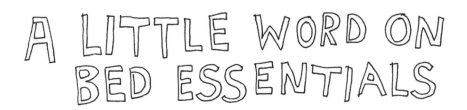

A LITTLE WORD ON BED ESSENTIALS

 SOME DAYS you might not have the energy to concentrate on reading lots of words. At such times picture books can be particularly comforting, whisking you away with their magical imagery.

 LAVENDER PILLOW MIST is a wonderful bedside essential. For many years the scent of the lavender flower has been used for therapeutic purposes, encouraging relaxation and aiding restful sleep. A few little sprays on your pillow should do the trick.

 IN THE COLDER MONTHS a pair of woolly bed socks can make feet heavenly warm … hand-knitted by nanna or those old favourites with the holes … cosy is priority!

 TEA IS A PROVEN soothing agent! When tucking in try caffeine-free types like rooibos, chamomile (very sleep-inducing!), peppermint, or special 'sleepy time' blends. When seeking refreshment try re-energising blends with citrus flavours or a light, fragrant green tea.

 'JOURNALING' is an essential tucked-in art form. Use your personal journal to record your ideas, spill out your good, bad or in-between thoughts, draw things you see and imagine, remember your dreams, collect things like tickets, cards or newspaper cut-outs, and make every day worth it by acknowledging the small but marvellous things that tickle your heart. For more on the therapeutic benefits of journaling turn to page 99.

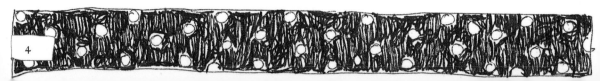

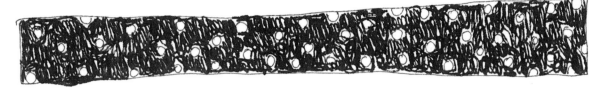

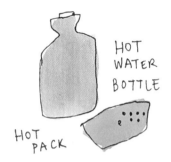

HOT WATER BOTTLE

HOT PACK

GREAT FOR CRAMPS, aches and pains, even chilly feet in winter, is the hot water bottle, or heat pack. The natural pain-fighting wonders of simple heat can't be underestimated. Just make sure the water isn't boiling, that you release the air before sealing and that the cap is screwed on nice and tight.

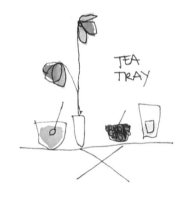

TEA TRAY

FOR TUCKED-IN dining comfort and convenience, a good tea tray is essential! See the 'Preparing a Tea Tray' on page 85 in the Nurturing section, along with some comfort food recipes to nourish your body and soul.

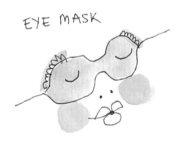

EYE MASK

FOR DAYTIME SIESTAS, aeroplanes, light bedrooms, shift workers and migraine sufferers, an eye mask is a good investment. Glamorous silk varieties make you feel less pirate and more princess.

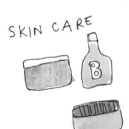

SKIN CARE

KEEPING YOUR skin hydrated and refreshed can make you feel instantly brighter. Deliciously natural body lotions and potions should be part of your tucked-in ritual showing your body love, care and a bit of pampering.

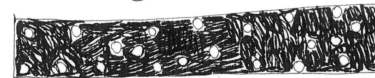

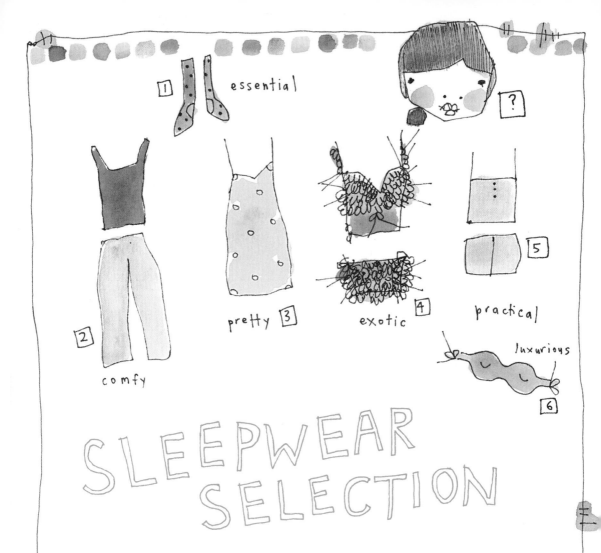

1 essential

?

2 comfy

pretty 3

exotic 4

practical 5

luxurious 6

SLEEPWEAR SELECTION

When tucking into a fresh, clean and cosy bed it is essential to ensure your 'bedwear' is also optimally comfortable. There is a wonderful world of sleepwear available for your tucking-in needs, indeed there is so much choice it may be hard to discern what to select! Options range from the comfy to the pretty, the exotic to the practical; from the slipper to the Ugg to the unusual socks with compartmentalised toe options. Sleepwear selection is not only a crucial part of your sleeping preparation and comfort, it is a seasonal art and must be undertaken with a degree of sensitivity.

On the next page are some signs to look out for that indicate bad bedwear.

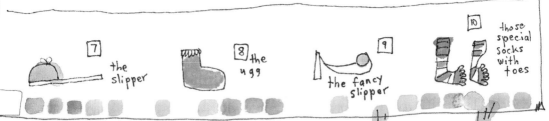

7 the slipper

8 the ugg

9 the fancy slipper

10 those special socks with toes

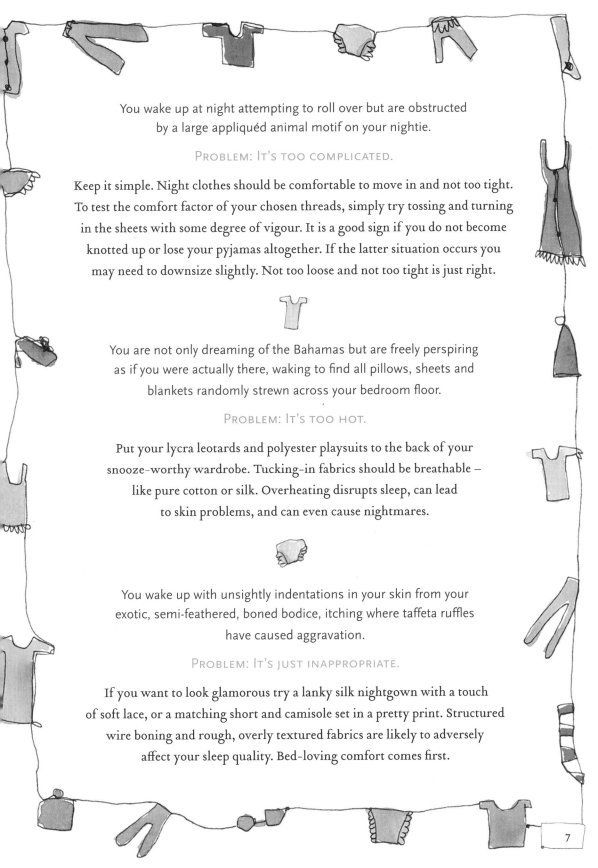

You wake up at night attempting to roll over but are obstructed
by a large appliquéd animal motif on your nightie.

Problem: It's too complicated.

Keep it simple. Night clothes should be comfortable to move in and not too tight.
To test the comfort factor of your chosen threads, simply try tossing and turning
in the sheets with some degree of vigour. It is a good sign if you do not become
knotted up or lose your pyjamas altogether. If the latter situation occurs you
may need to downsize slightly. Not too loose and not too tight is just right.

You are not only dreaming of the Bahamas but are freely perspiring
as if you were actually there, waking to find all pillows, sheets and
blankets randomly strewn across your bedroom floor.

Problem: It's too hot.

Put your lycra leotards and polyester playsuits to the back of your
snooze-worthy wardrobe. Tucking-in fabrics should be breathable –
like pure cotton or silk. Overheating disrupts sleep, can lead
to skin problems, and can even cause nightmares.

You wake up with unsightly indentations in your skin from your
exotic, semi-feathered, boned bodice, itching where taffeta ruffles
have caused aggravation.

Problem: It's just inappropriate.

If you want to look glamorous try a lanky silk nightgown with a touch
of soft lace, or a matching short and camisole set in a pretty print. Structured
wire boning and rough, overly textured fabrics are likely to adversely
affect your sleep quality. Bed-loving comfort comes first.

CHOOSE YOUR SLEEPING CAP

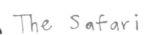

The Safari

A little bit adventurous?
Why not sign up for a safari while you snooze with this unique sleeping cap option? Be whisked away on a wild adventure dream or two for an invigorating and memorable night's slumber. Monsieur Stripes is an expert guide with impressive local knowledge.

The Evening Primrose

For those partial to florals and charmed by the miracle of nature encapsulated in this very special blossom, this is the sleeping cap for you. When dark falls the wonderful evening primrose releases its delightful perfume, infusing your dreams with sweetness.

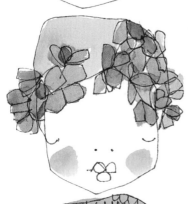

The Woolly

For those in cool climates, battling head colds or simply wishing to keep cosy, The Woolly, with its built-in ear warmers, is for you. Especially magic and warming when hand knitted with love.

The Lullaby

Falling asleep to beautiful music is soothing and luxurious. Music can help to transport us into our dreams. Experience rhythms, sounds and vibrations delivered straight to your ears by The Lullaby's built-in earphones. Sure to enchant, its menu of musical options will suit even the most discerning sleeper.

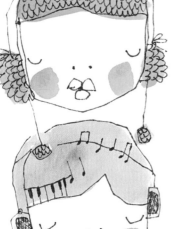

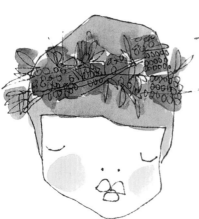

The Lavender Bush

Stressed? Restless? Exhausted?
Anticipating deep and wonderful sleep?

The Lavender Bush is more tiara than sleeping cap, but contributes greatly to making your slumber even more nourishing.

Weave some lavender through your hair and experience its famously therapeutic qualities.

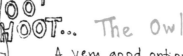

The Swan Lake

Dreaming of dancing but suffering from two left feet? Well... IN YOUR DREAMS! Let Ms Swan guide you through a whimsical world of tutus, twists and turns, velvet curtains, applause, suspense and anticipation. Live and breathe the moment, feel the magic, and wake to feel nimble and utterly inspired!

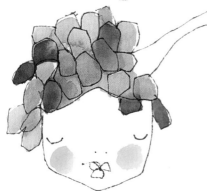

HOOT HOOT... The Owl

A very good option for those wanting to keep an eye on things even when taking 40 winks. This little fellow will guarantee to look out for you all night through.

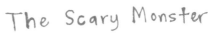

The Scary Monster

Especially for those scared of the dark is The Scary Monster, who is sure to scare off any nasties. For a safe and restful sleep he is always a good and sensible choice.

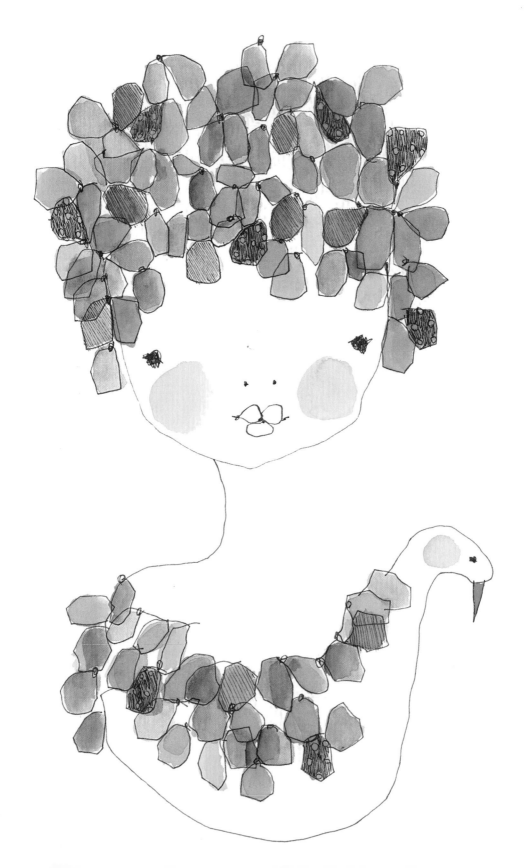

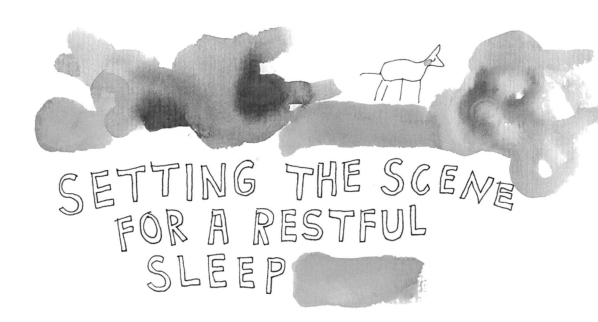

SETTING THE SCENE FOR A RESTFUL SLEEP

SETTING THE SCENE FOR A RESTFUL SLEEP
INVOLVES CREATING A DIVINE, CALM SANCTUARY
IN WHICH TO SLUMBER, DREAM, RELAX AND WAKE.

With consideration for all your senses — what you see,
what you touch, what you hear, what you smell and even
what you taste — you will be able to create a sleeping space to
comfort and nurture you while expressing your creativity.

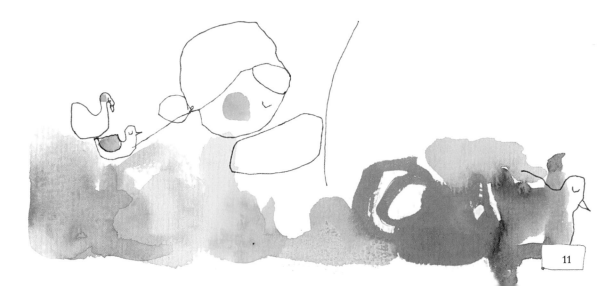

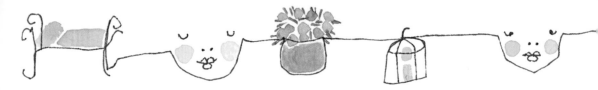

SEE YOUR BEDROOM should contain things that you enjoy looking at, such as artworks, special ornaments, beautiful flowers or cherished photographs. Our tastes are so varied and unique, and creating a bedroom haven that feels right is very personal. Simply ensure that when you are horizontal you can look around and be uplifted by things in which you see beauty. If you have a window to the outside world, organise your furniture so you can enjoy the experience of being tucked in cosily whilst watching the outdoor rhythms of night and day. Take pleasure in the changing sky, the dancing trees, the cheeky birds or simply the way the light moves and creates shadows.

NATURAL LIGHT IN the bedroom during daytime hours is optimal, but if you are using artificial lighting make sure it is subtle and unobtrusive. At night, ensure that your room is dark enough and that streetlights or other light sources are blocked out. If you are getting too much light at night, you are likely to confuse your body's internal clock, making sleep more difficult and compromising its quality. Ideal sleep conditions are dark, quiet and cool. Use block-out blinds, eye masks or heavy drapes to block out unwanted light.

Colour has a profound effect in creating a relaxing interior. Powder blues, soft wheat and sage-green tones are said to create a calming effect, while bold yellows, reds or oranges are known to overstimulate. Lighter colours can brighten a dark room and make small spaces seem larger, while darker tones tend to achieve the opposite effect. Selecting paint colours for your bedroom walls is an art; it might take a few attempts to get it right but it is worth taking your time to see a wonderful result.

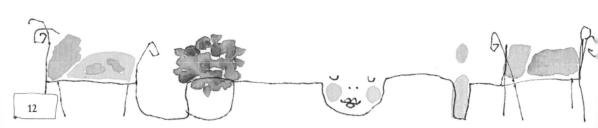

TOUCH

YOUR SLEEPING SPACE should be full of textures that make you feel good: fresh cotton sheets, a heavenly mattress, pillows you can melt into, a snug mohair blanket in winter, soft comfy pyjamas or a delicate silky nightgown. Try cosy rugs underfoot if you're feeling chilly, or a good pair of knitted socks to warm cold feet. Other lovely textures can be found in furniture: smooth cool wood or the worn, well-loved upholstery of your favourite armchair. When your space feels good, you are bound to feel good too.

HEAR

THE SOUND ENVIRONMENT in your sleeping space should be in tune with your mood and not cause any disturbance to your rest. In the mornings you might listen to lively music to transport and inspire you, while gentle evening music might relax you and help you unwind at the end of your day. Lullabies are wonderful songs for the sleeping space. You can find a series of lullabies and their stories on pages 46–53. These enchanting, whimsical pieces of sleep music are examples of lullabies that appeal to young and old hearts alike.

Environmental noise that is beyond your control might be disruptive to your rest. If you live on a noisy street, near loud neighbours, under a flight path, or in any other space where noise becomes an issue, you might like to try a few measures to ensure the disturbance is kept to a minimum.

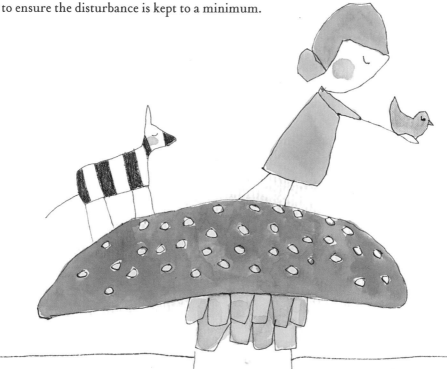

The gentle, constant hum of a fan can often block out surrounding noise and is an option worth trying, as are silicone ear plugs, which are comfortable and effective sound blockers. Investing in an indoor water feature or playing very gentle music through the night might also detract from unwanted noise, providing it isn't more of a distraction. Loud ticking clocks, televisions and ringing phones are harsh sounds that should ideally be kept out of your sleeping space. Shocking alarm clocks should also be avoided. Opt instead for a gentler wake-up call, such as music from your favourite radio station, or ask a responsible family member or pet to wake you at a suitable hour. The first moments of your day are quite special and should be treated with care.

SMELL

SWEET-SMELLING FLOWERS, naturally scented candles, gentle incense or the fragrance of essential oil infusing your sleeping space can really help to set the mood. Smells can be rich and magical. Certain scents can bring back vivid memories and transport us to other times and places; others may invigorate us or help us wind down. Ensure that your choice of fragrances reflects your mood, and is in no way overpowering.

Certain scents are particularly fitting for your bedroom and help to create a suitable atmosphere. Chamomile, neroli and rose are relaxing, floral aromas that calm the mind and create a sense of harmony and balance. Ylang ylang, vanilla, frankincense, clary sage and lavender are also wonderful bedroom fragrances. A few drops of lavender oil on your pillow or a bunch of freshly cut lavender

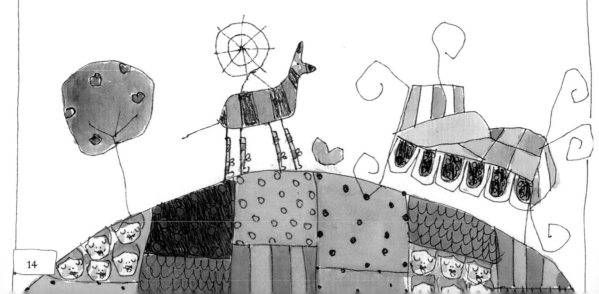

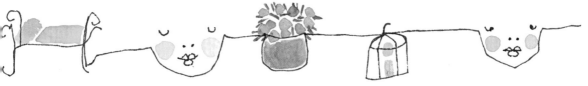

on your bedside table make very soothing additions to your sleeping space. If insects bother you in the night, a few drops of lavender oil on your curtains can keep them at bay. Jasmine is also ideal in the bedroom – it is a wonderful, relaxing fragrance said to treat anxiety and depression. By planting a jasmine plant outside your bedroom window you can enjoy the enchanting night-time fragrance of the blossom.

TASTE WHILE SOME EXPERTS recommend keeping food out of the bedroom, when we are unwell or feeling exhausted, 'tucked-in dining' provides an opportunity to indulge in comfort foods that make us smile from the inside out. Certain homemade wonders simply taste better when tucked in: a warm cup of tea, a sweet almond biscuit, or a heart-warming bowl of vegetable soup. Take a look at the Sleepy Supermarket Trolley section on pages 54–57 for some tips on foods that induce sleepiness, or try some of the comfort-food recipes on pages 86–93. Investing in a good tea tray also makes for an indulgent, comfortable tucked-in dining experience!

LAST BUT NOT LEAST, make sure that your bedroom is an indulgent haven, not a multi-tasking area in which you work as well as rest. Banning computers, mobile phones and work documents is highly recommended, as they only bring your day-to-day stress into your sacred space. It is very important psychologically to distinguish between your sleeping/dreaming life and your working life, knowing that stepping into your bedroom means unwinding and recharging your mind and body in peace and quiet. Once you have given your private sleeping sanctuary a little bit of TLC, simply lie back, relax and enjoy the wonderful atmosphere that you have created. Take pride in caring for your special space and allow it to enrich your days and your senses.

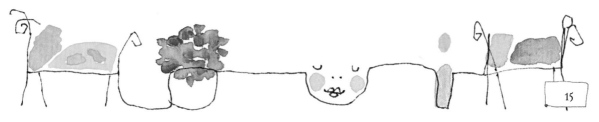

THE SOOTHING MAGIC OF A GOOD BATH

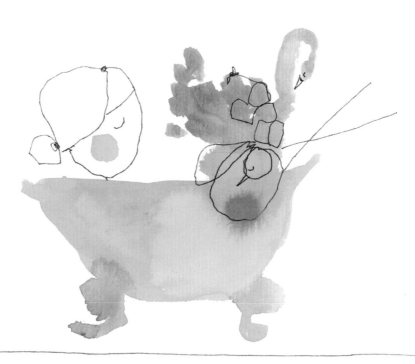

BATHING HAS A RICH AND FASCINATING HISTORY OF CREATING LUXURY FOR THE SENSES, SOOTHING THE MIND AND BODY, AND PROMOTING WELLBEING. WHY NOT LET BATHING BECOME A RELAXING PART OF YOUR SLEEP-LOVING ROUTINE?

As early as 2000 BC Ancient Egyptians bathed in natural craters in the earth's surface, filled with water and warmed by burning rocks. Egyptian royalty were later known to bathe with essential oils and flowers, exploring the richness of aromatherapy long before our time. Our Ancient Greek and Roman ancestors celebrated a vibrant, social bathing culture. Early baths, usually constructed near naturally occurring hot springs, offered therapeutic rewards to health-conscious bathers: a combination of heat and water to soothe sore muscles and relax the body, steam to invigorate the skin, perfumes to enliven the senses, and massage to untie inner knots.

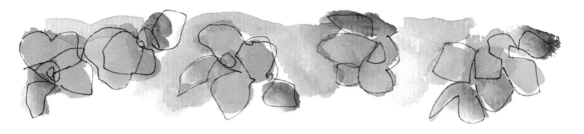

ACCORDING TO THE ANCIENT GREEK PHYSICIAN HIPPOCRATES, a perfumed bath and scented massage every day is the way to good health. Indeed, in the classical world, bathing was considered as beneficial for mental health as it was for physical wellbeing. Public baths quickly became hubs for social interaction, not just for cleansing and relaxation. The Ancient Romans even designed and constructed elaborate, beautiful buildings dedicated to public bathing, fitted with statues, grand lecture halls and libraries. Within the walls of these thermae our bathing ancestors would remove dirt and grease from their bodies before moving through rooms of varying temperatures and indulging in perfumed oil massages. Afterwards they could stroll in the gardens, attend literary recitals, watch jugglers or acrobats, or visit the library. How's that for indulgence?

A CONNECTION BETWEEN BATHING and wellness in daily life has also been long celebrated in Asia. Fragrant wooden bathtubs, usually made from cedar, are central to the Japanese tradition, in which the natural oils of the wood imbue the warm bath water with a delicate, vitalising scent. The Yuya hot springs in the city of Shinshiro, Japan have a history spanning 1200 years. They are located in the quiet valley of the Itajiki River, and it's believed the waters can cure many ailments. There is an old story that tells of a legendary monk named Rishu who flew in on the wind to bathe here.

In the time of the Ottoman Empire in Turkey, the hamam (sauna/bath) was a place where people would not only bathe but also where marvellous social gatherings would take place, often involving feasts and dancing. Ceremonies before weddings, celebrations for newborn babies, parties for high holidays or simply pure beautification, were all part of Turkish bathing culture.

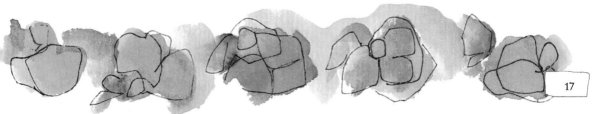

N THE EARLY DAYS, baths were infused with bundles of herbs or flowers wrapped in muslin. Today, many varieties of bath salts, powders and oils are available to scent and enhance baths. Pure organic essential oils diluted in a vegetable oil carrier may also be used to perfume your bath. Essential oils must be used with care however, as certain varieties such as basil, cinnamon, clove, peppermint, thyme and ginger can irritate sensitive skin and should be used minimally, if at all. Their vapour can really sting if it gets in your eyes, so be careful. Some scents such as pennyroyal, nutmeg, rosemary, basil, jasmine, sage and juniper berry are not appropriate during pregnancy either, or if you are using certain medications. Any essential oils must be used sparingly during pregnancy. It is best to check with your doctor if you have any doubts.

GRAPEFRUIT AND LAVENDER are two very safe oils to use: lavender is best for the evening, to soothe tired muscles and promote restful sleep, while grapefruit is an energising scent which can be used to enliven your senses as you take a morning bath. If you are experiencing muscle pain, marjoram might be your oil of choice. Fill the bath with warm water, dilute 6–8 drops of the oil in a tablespoon of vegetable, grapeseed or sweet almond oil and sprinkle on to the surface of the water. Don't forget to close the door so those wonderful vapours don't escape! You might lie back with a book, some beautiful music, or the light of a glowing candle – whatever makes you feel at ease. Bathing for a minimum of ten minutes is recommended, but if you have the time for a good half-hour soak then just relax, indulge and enjoy.

Apart from drawing on essential oils, there are many simple and creative ways to add spice to your bathing life. Chamomile tea bags infused in a bath soothe skin complaints and counter insomnia, while green teabags detoxify. Adding orange or lemon peel to your bath, or even sprigs of rosemary, makes for a fresh and stimulating aromatic experience. Bergamot is another stimulating fragrance suitable for a morning bath.

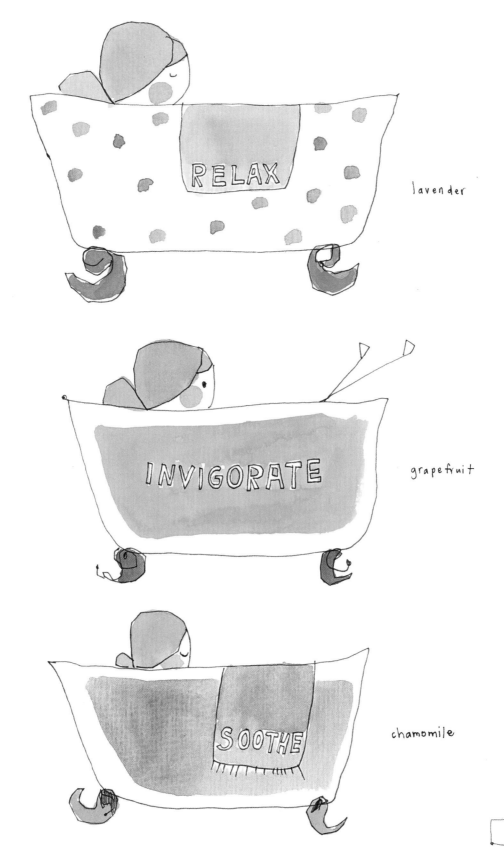

lavender

grapefruit

chamomile

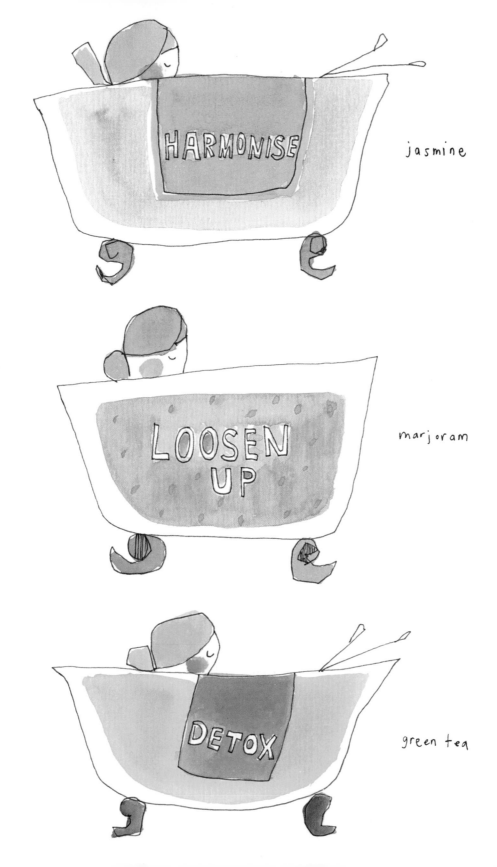

HARMONISE

jasmine

LOOSEN UP

marjoram

DETOX

green tea

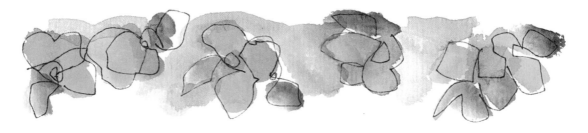

FOR RASHES, BITES, ITCHING, ECZEMA and other skin conditions try an oatmeal bath (as long as you aren't allergic to gluten). Simply use a blender or food processor to grind a cupful of ordinary breakfast oats to a fine powder. Add the powder to your warm bath water, stirring well to remove any clumps. You can soak for 15–20 minutes in your oat bath, twice a day or as required, allowing your skin to settle and regenerate. A gluten-free alternative is a goat milk bath. Add one and a half cups of goat milk powder (available from health food shops) to your bath to soften and nourish skin. Goat milk is very gentle on sensitive skin and has a lovely sweet, milky scent. Once you emerge from the water, pat your skin dry with a soft towel rather than rubbing and further aggravating sensitivities.

IF YOU ARE WITHOUT A BATHTUB AND FEELING WOEFUL, all is not lost! You can still reap the full mind-and-body benefits of aromatic bathing, even without a tub. There is an extensive range of positively magnificent shower oils and gels available which can be applied to the skin with a soft, lightly textured sponge during showering. Some varieties will even exfoliate as well as leave you smelling divine! And instead of immersing yourself in scented water you might like to burn essential oils in your bathroom as you shower and perform your bathing routine. Simply add a few drops of essential oil to a little water warmed over a tea-light candle oil burner. You may otherwise opt for a scented candle to infuse your bathroom with your chosen scent.

Just remember to pay attention to fragrance combinations, be careful with very potent oils and try to avoid clashing or overpowering scents in your bathroom. The soothing magic of hot water against skin works wonders on tired, sore bodies. Turn bathing into a daily luxury with a touch of creativity, care and inspiration.

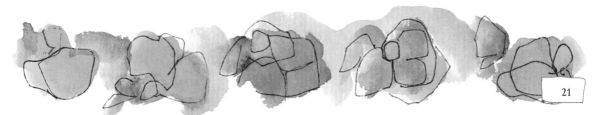

SHADOW PUPPETRY

The ancient and accessible art of shadow puppetry can become part of your tucking-in experience! With a bit of wall and a pinch of light, see creatures take shape and come alive in your very own bedroom!

scene one

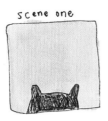

scene two

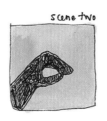

scene three

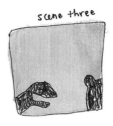

SHADOW PUPPETRY is a richly creative art form with a most unusual history. More than 2000 years ago in China, a minister of the Emperor Wu noticed the wonderful shadows created on the walls when children played with their dolls. He also noticed that Emperor Wu, riddled with despair and sadness following the death of his favourite concubine, needed some serious uplifting. The minister conceived of the idea to create a shadow puppet representing his master's lost love. He hoped that this dancing, floating silhouette would reawaken the emperor's senses, and draw him from his depression.

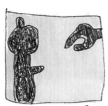

scene four

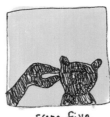

scene five

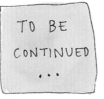

TO BE CONTINUED ...

scene six

N Emperor Wu's day, shadow puppets were made from stretched donkey skins or dried sheepskins. The cut-out forms were placed before a light source and projected through a sheet, causing the shadows to appear clearly to an audience on the other side. The movement of the puppets was controlled by strings attached to rods, the puppeteer typically using one hand to control the puppet's neck and the other hand to manipulate its wrists. Translucent colour was sometimes fitted into the cut-out shape, with overlapping forms and crossing colours making for interesting shadow play. With a combination of music, moving image, colour and sound effects, shadow puppet shows provided engaging entertainment with an exciting sense of immediacy and playfulness.

Shadow puppetry was also popular in Europe. Live theatre declined following the fall of the Roman Empire, but travelling puppeteers kept the theatrical tradition alive and carried the craft into new creative and geographical territory.

Shadow puppetry has been illuminating and entertaining audiences over the centuries, playing a part in religious teaching and even political parody. The simplicity and beauty of the craft continues to delight young and old hearts around the world. Java, Turkey and India boast particularly rich traditions of shadow puppetry.

Today puppets are seldom made from animal hides; instead, paper, cardboard, wood and recycled household objects are ideal materials for making our own puppets. More intricate puppets are constructed with strings, but simpler puppets without joints can be attached to single rods controlled by hand. While the range of movement is compromised, the essence of the moving shapes and colours remains the same. In some performances sheets are used through which the shadows are projected, but a wall alone will suffice. By correctly angling your bedside lamp on to your wall you will be able to see your puppets' shadows come to life directly. Just ensure that you, the puppeteer, are located between the light source and the shadow surface.

HOW TO MAKE YOUR OWN 'TUCKED IN' PUPPET SHOW

SHADOW PUPPETS MAKE FOR PERFECT TUCKED-IN ENTERTAINMENT.
In the cosy atmosphere of your dimly lit room, and in the comfort of your own bed, you can make stories come to life and dance across your walls in shadow form. While different shadow shapes can be made by simply using your hands, below you will find a guide to hand-making original puppets with which to play.

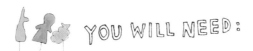 YOU WILL NEED:

- Paper, cardboard, recycled household objects such as egg cartons, toilet rolls, or any other lightweight objects you can use to make interesting shadows
- Pencils and pens to trace forms
- A stick or rod to hold up your puppet
- Scissors
- Glue and sticky tape
- Wires and brass paper fasteners for joint movement (for more complex puppets)
- Coloured cellophane to insert into puppet cut-outs for a 'stained glass' effect
- A light source, such as a bedside lamp, lantern or candle
- A blank screen or a wall upon which to project

1. Brainstorm your puppet's character, personality and story. Remember that you have free rein to create your characters, as well as the props and scenery to accompany them. Would you like them to be human or animal forms, plants, inanimate objects or buildings? Are you creating a mystery, a fairytale, or some other kind of night-time story? Will your puppets dance and sing? Are they cheeky, energetic or shy? The possibilities are endless – let your creativity run wild. Music, fairytales, or real-life events might inspire your puppet's stories.

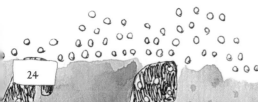

2 Create your puppet forms. Draw your chosen shapes directly on to your cardboard and cut them out. Inserting pieces of coloured cellophane into your figures will create a wonderful, stained-glass effect.

3 Create movement. You can create additional movement by using brass paper fasteners and wire to create shoulder, elbow, wrist, knee and ankle joints, attaching rods to those limbs to control movement. Alternatively, simply fixing a stick or rod to the back of your puppet will suffice. Ensure that your puppet is well fixed to its stick – this will prevent any nasty falls or embarrassing disappearances mid-performance!

4 Choose your surface. Make sure your wall is empty so that your show space is unobstructed. Obstructions will interfere with the visibility of your shadows. If you are tucked in you may like to choose the wall next to your bed.

5 Let there be light! Select a light source like a bedside lamp, a spotlight or a candle. While a stronger light source is ideal, if using candlelight simply ensure that all background light is dimmed for optimum visibility. Angle the light over your head to minimise extra shadows and ensure you are positioned between the light source and the wall.

6 Showtime! Now you can bring your story and characters to life in shadow form, with the added accompaniments of background music and sound effects if you so desire. Two or more pairs of hands will allow for more characters onstage at once, so if you have a partner in crime, or an enthusiastic audience member, perhaps you could draw on their creative contribution as well.

Now just snuggle back, relax, and enjoy the magic of
your wonderful homemade theatre!

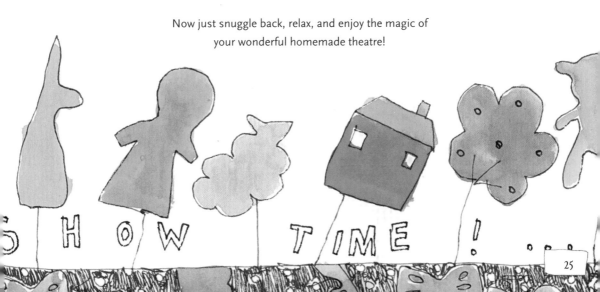

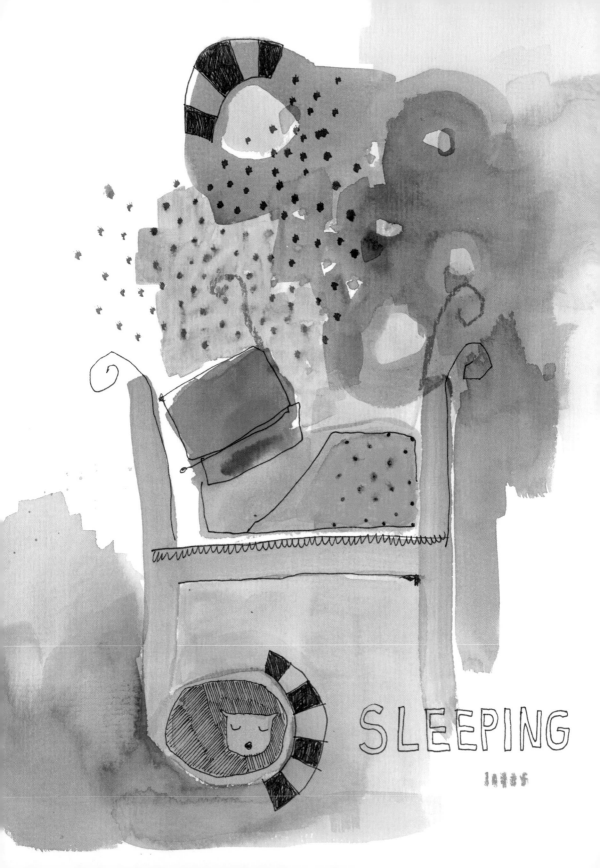

BED, HAMMOCK, TENT OR IGLOO?

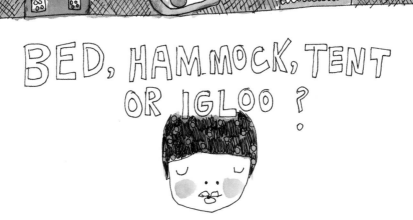

Where do you tuck in at night?

MANY OF US have beds in which to snuggle, but all around the world people sleep in all sorts of different locations and 'tuck in' in various ways.

Eskimos snooze in their igloos, campers get cosy in tents and travellers on the sea take forty winks in houseboats, submarines or cruise-ship cabins. Explorers might tuck in to cosy caves while astronauts sleep vertically in spaceships, tethered to something fixed so they can't drift around the craft.

Sleeping styles can be culturally specific and moulded by customs, traditions and circumstance. In hot tropical climates some people tuck in to hammocks under the stars, simple seaside huts or breezy tree houses. In other countries around the world families sleep together in one-room shelters which also incorporate eating and bathing areas.

Tatami mats have a special place in Japanese sleeping culture. Woven from rice straw, *tatami* traditionally measure three by six feet and are three inches thick. Rather than upright beds with frames, *tatami* mats accommodate sleeping at ground level. The layout of the *tatami* on the floor is a precise art; an inappropriate arrangement of the matting is said to be highly inauspicious.

There are reports of people falling asleep in all sorts of peculiar places: ATM booths, laundromats, even supermarkets! You might like to look through these pictures and mark in the little boxes where you have or haven't slept – bunk bed, caravan or cubby house?

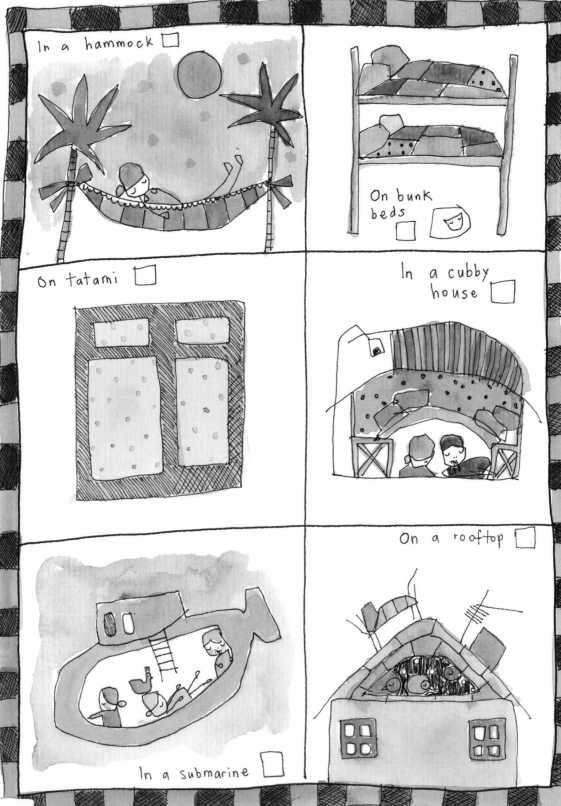

In a hammock ☐

On bunk beds ☐

On tatami ☐

In a cubby house ☐

In a submarine ☐

On a rooftop ☐

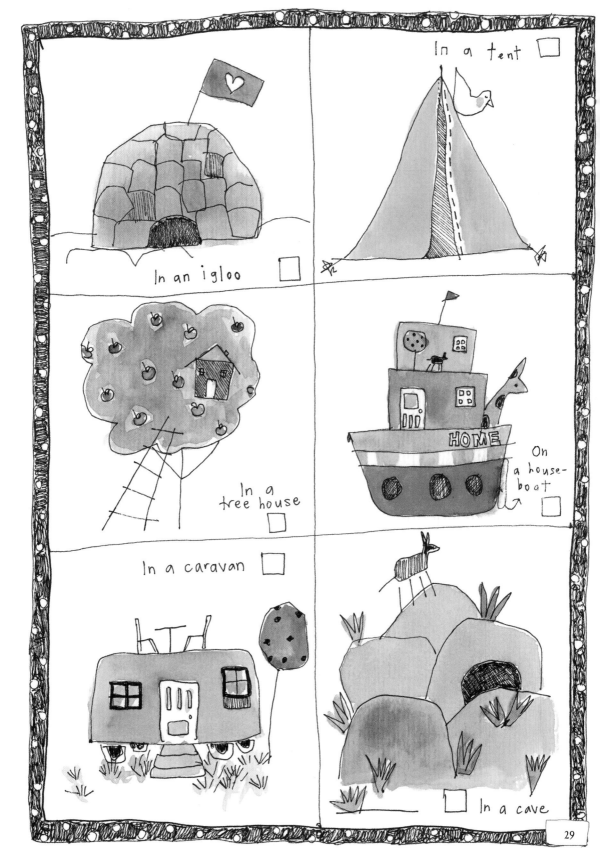

In a tent ☐

In an igloo ☐

In a tree house ☐

On a house-boat ☐

In a caravan ☐

In a cave ☐

WHAT DOES YOUR SLEEPING POSITION SAY ABOUT YOUR PERSONALITY?

THE 'SIDE KOALA'

You ENJOY brunch on Sundays and hand-knitted jumpers. You are affectionate, loyal and well-read. Like most side koalas, you thrive in intelligent company.

THE 'UNDER THE BED'

Possibly ECCENTRIC, you built impressive cubby houses as a child and have a penchant for caves. Your particular interests include the history of the Roman catacombs and the hidden treasures of Ancient Egypt.

THE COUCH

You HARBOUR a particular fondness for television. The likelihood of stale popcorn being found between your couch and your cushions is extremely high, as are remote control 'pillow marks' on your cheek, particularly on Monday mornings.

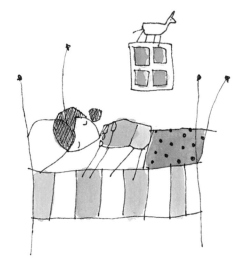

THE SIDE KOALA

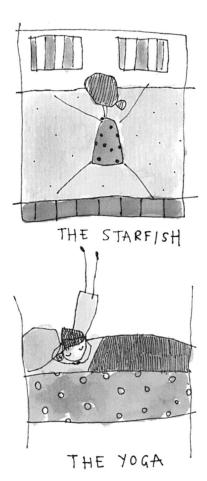

THE STARFISH

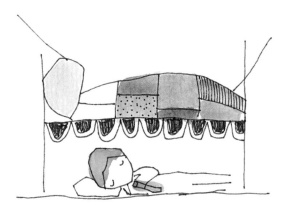

THE 'UNDER THE BED'

THE YOGA

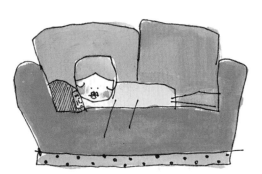

THE COUCH

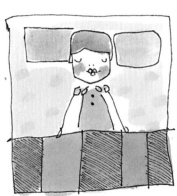

THE SUNNY SIDE UP

THE STARFISH

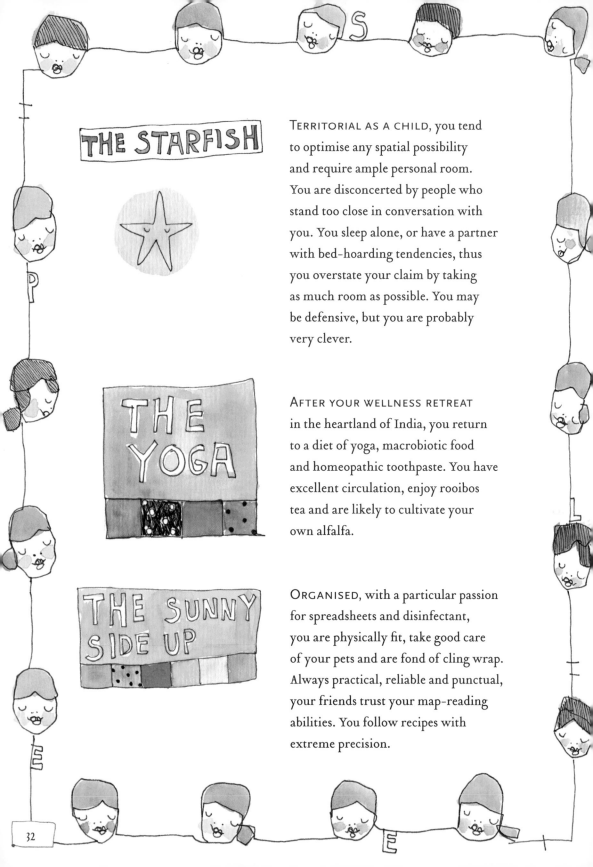

TERRITORIAL AS A CHILD, you tend to optimise any spatial possibility and require ample personal room. You are disconcerted by people who stand too close in conversation with you. You sleep alone, or have a partner with bed-hoarding tendencies, thus you overstate your claim by taking as much room as possible. You may be defensive, but you are probably very clever.

THE YOGA

AFTER YOUR WELLNESS RETREAT in the heartland of India, you return to a diet of yoga, macrobiotic food and homeopathic toothpaste. You have excellent circulation, enjoy rooibos tea and are likely to cultivate your own alfalfa.

THE SUNNY SIDE UP

ORGANISED, with a particular passion for spreadsheets and disinfectant, you are physically fit, take good care of your pets and are fond of cling wrap. Always practical, reliable and punctual, your friends trust your map-reading abilities. You follow recipes with extreme precision.

COUNTING SHEEP...

IF THE AGE-OLD PRACTICE OF COUNTING SHEEP DOESN'T SEND YOU INTO A DREAMY SLUMBER, YOU MIGHT FANCY TAKING ON THIS CHALLENGE.

It goes without saying that sleep doesn't always come easily, but with a bit of imagination, a giggle, and a few sheep, we might all stand a better chance of discovering heavenly rest! The following 'sheep directory' will introduce you to a flock of unique and individual sheep, each with his or her own occupation and secret passion. Your job is to memorise each sheep in order and in detail. By the time you accomplish this feat you should be extremely weary, if not already fast asleep!

Get ready to meet and greet your new woolly friends.

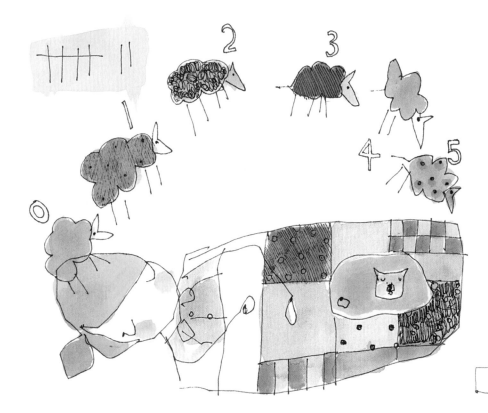

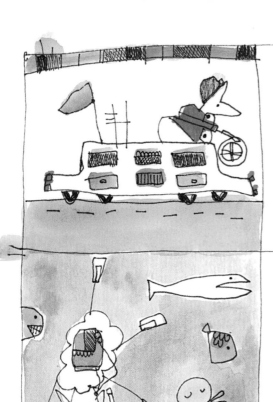

Name : Ferdinand Esquire

Profession: Stretch Limousine Chauffeur

Favourite thing: Glow in the dark putt putt golf

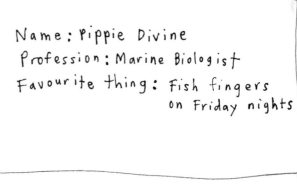

Name: Pippie Divine

Profession: Marine Biologist

Favourite thing: Fish fingers on Friday nights

Name : Gomez Gonzales

Profession: Private Detective

Favourite thing: Film noir

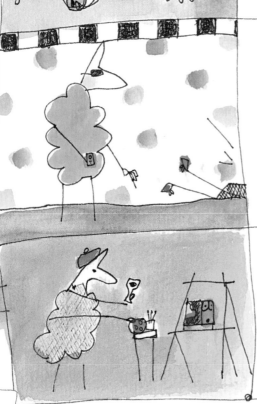

Name: Francoise laPom Pom

Profession: Artist

Favourite thing: Vino rosso and/or Debussy

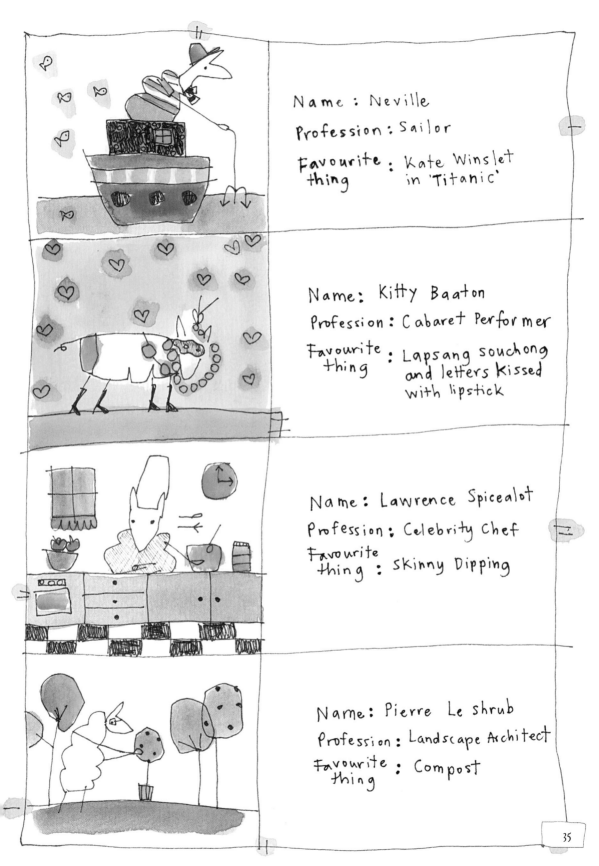

Name : Neville
Profession : Sailor
Favourite thing : Kate Winslet in 'Titanic'

Name: Kitty Baaton
Profession : Cabaret Performer
Favourite thing : Lapsang souchong and letters kissed with lipstick

Name : Lawrence Spicealot
Profession : Celebrity Chef
Favourite thing : Skinny Dipping

Name: Pierre Le shrub
Profession : Landscape Architect
Favourite thing : Compost

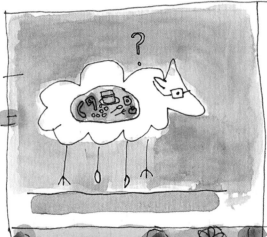

Name: Bob

Profession: Food Critic

Favourite thing: Peruvian Duck with wild rice; side of rocket, pear and Hazelnut salad, then profiteroles (secret truth: honey on toast)

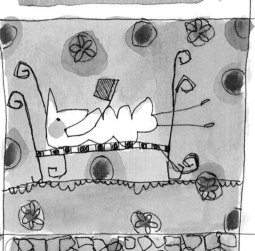

Name: Carmellina

Profession: Psychologist

Favourite thing: Jane Austen in bed

Name: Xander Thunderbolt

Profession: Champion Rock climber

Favourite thing: Chocolate chip biscuits with warm milk & honey

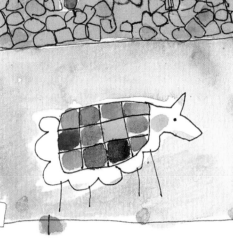

Name: Sabina stitch

Profession: Textile Designer

Favourite thing: Her walk-in doona-poncho

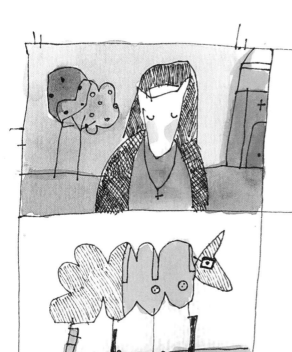

Name : Sister Delia Crumpet
Profession : Nun, choir master
Favourite thing: Choc tops
at the movies

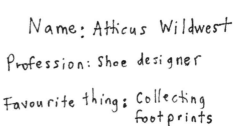

Name: Atticus Wildwest

Profession: Shoe designer

Favourite thing: Collecting
footprints

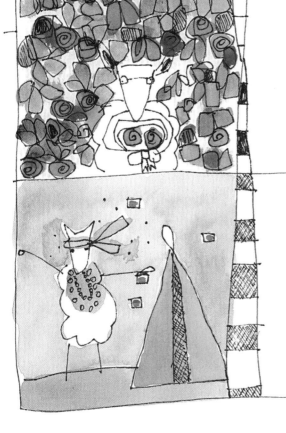

Name: Blossom Belle

Profession: Florist

Favourite thing: Blind
dating

Name: Sommerset Dupuy

Profession : Tarot reader

Favourite thing: Tofu
turkey
for Christmas
and/or Grandmother's
bead collection

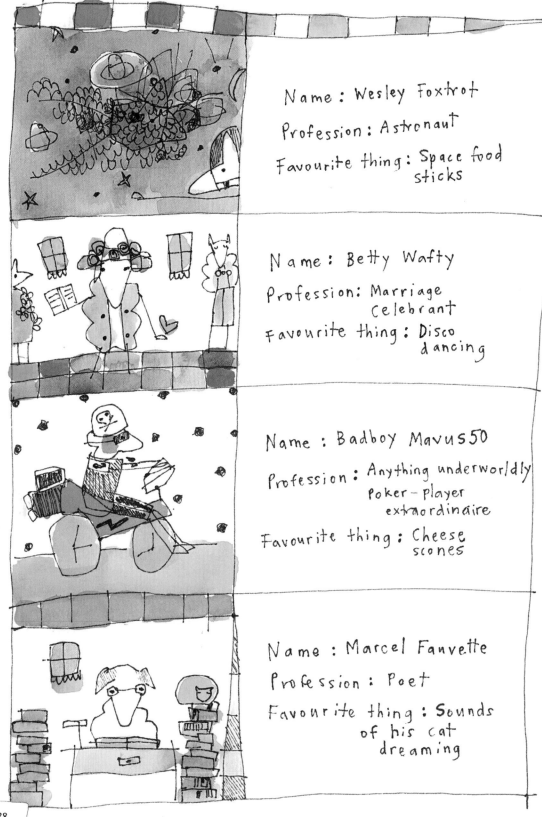

Name: Wesley Foxtrot

Profession: Astronaut

Favourite thing: Space food sticks

Name: Betty Wafty

Profession: Marriage Celebrant

Favourite thing: Disco dancing

Name: Badboy Mavus50

Profession: Anything underworldly Poker-player extraordinaire

Favourite thing: Cheese scones

Name: Marcel Fauvette

Profession: Poet

Favourite thing: Sounds of his cat dreaming

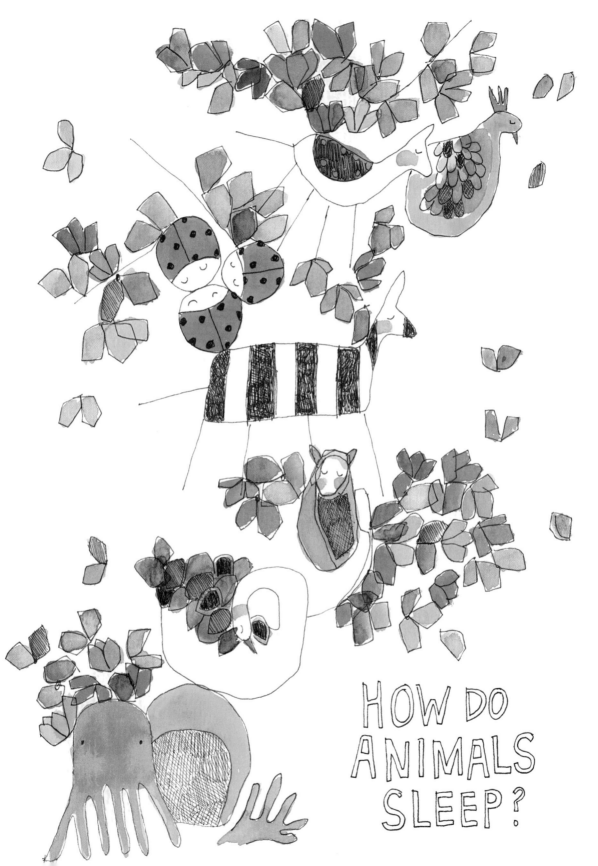

HOW DO
ANIMALS
SLEEP?

THE WEIRD AND WONDERFUL NIGHT LIFE OF OUR ANIMAL FRIENDS

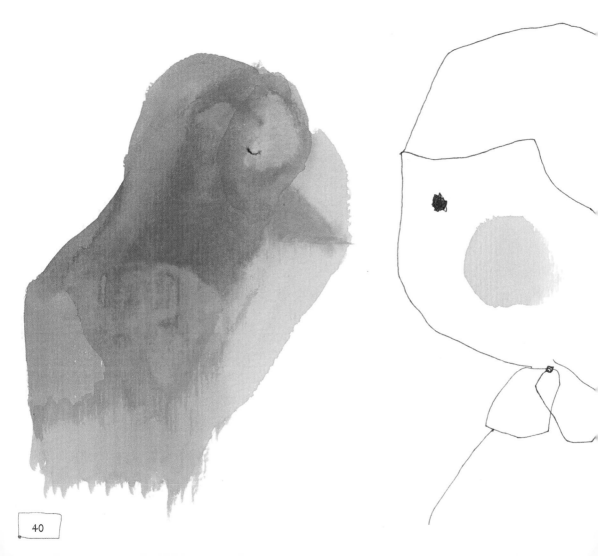

ANIMALS REQUIRE THE HEALING POWER OF SLEEP AS MUCH AS WE HUMAN BEINGS DO. DID YOU KNOW THAT EACH NIGHT WHILE YOU SLEEP COSILY IN YOUR BED THE LOGGERHEAD TURTLE IS 'SLEEP-SWIMMING' TO THE WATER'S SURFACE TO TAKE A BREATH HOURLY?

That sleepy octopi are seeking out underwater caves in which to spend the night, and that owls are busy creating plans, meeting friends and making music?

Welcome to the weird and wonderful nightlife of our animal friends! These next few pages celebrate and explore the sleeping antics of the various fauna with which we share our magical planet.

When you think you've got a lot on your mind and can't fall asleep, take a moment to think about the ducks, dolphins and flamingoes of this world that snooze with only half their brains asleep, watching out over their fellows and staying alert to potential environmental dangers. If you're feeling sleep deprived, spare a thought for the giraffe, whose sleeping time adds up to around a meagre 1.9 hours per day!

Whichever way you look at it – upside-down, lying down, eyes open wide or tightly shut – we all sleep. If our animal friends were to look at our human sleeping habits they would probably find us equally amusing. Take a moment to appreciate the uniqueness of the animals around you, and remember that we are all in this life together.

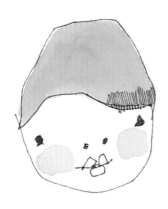
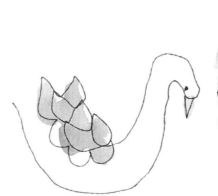
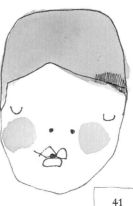

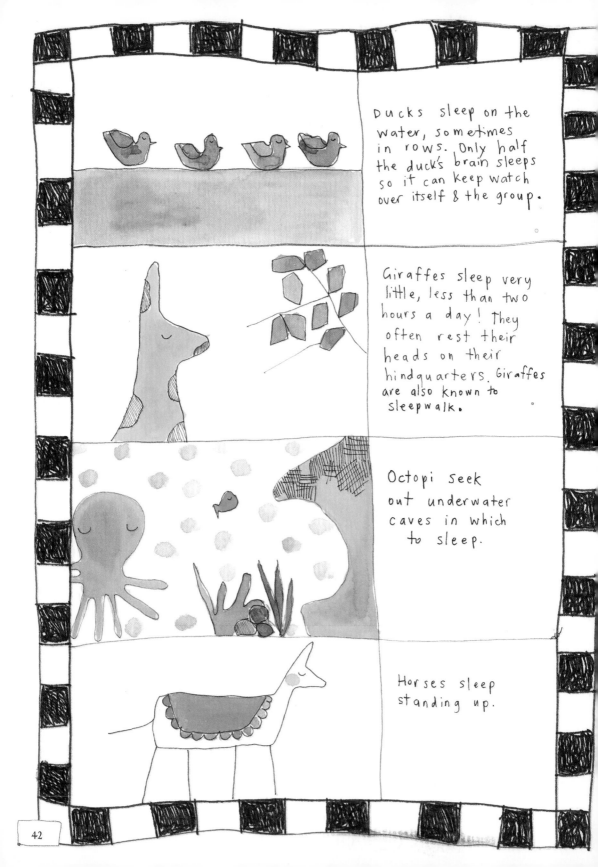

Ducks sleep on the water, sometimes in rows. Only half the duck's brain sleeps so it can keep watch over itself & the group.

Giraffes sleep very little, less than two hours a day! They often rest their heads on their hindquarters. Giraffes are also known to sleepwalk.

Octopi seek out underwater caves in which to sleep.

Horses sleep standing up.

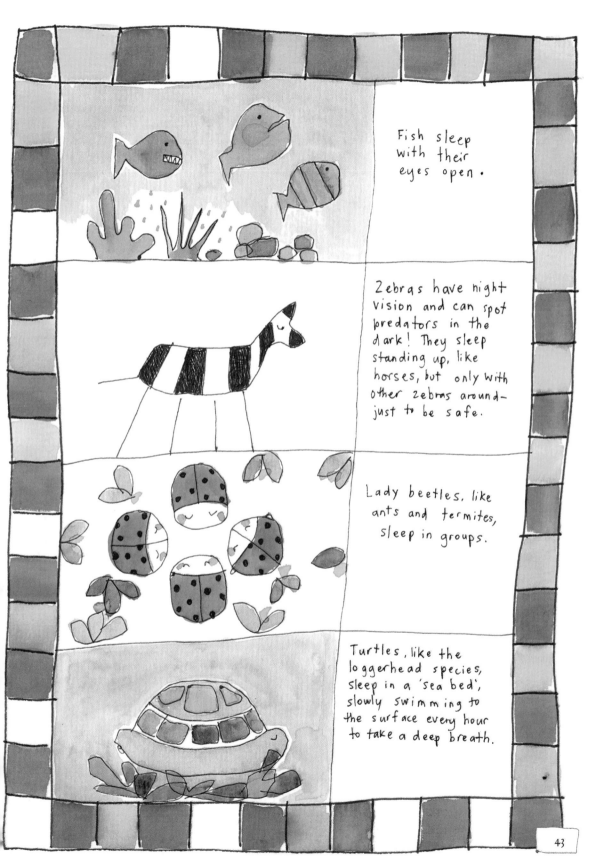

Fish sleep with their eyes open.

Zebras have night vision and can spot predators in the dark! They sleep standing up, like horses, but only with other zebras around — just to be safe.

Lady beetles, like ants and termites, sleep in groups.

Turtles, like the loggerhead species, sleep in a 'sea bed', slowly swimming to the surface every hour to take a deep breath.

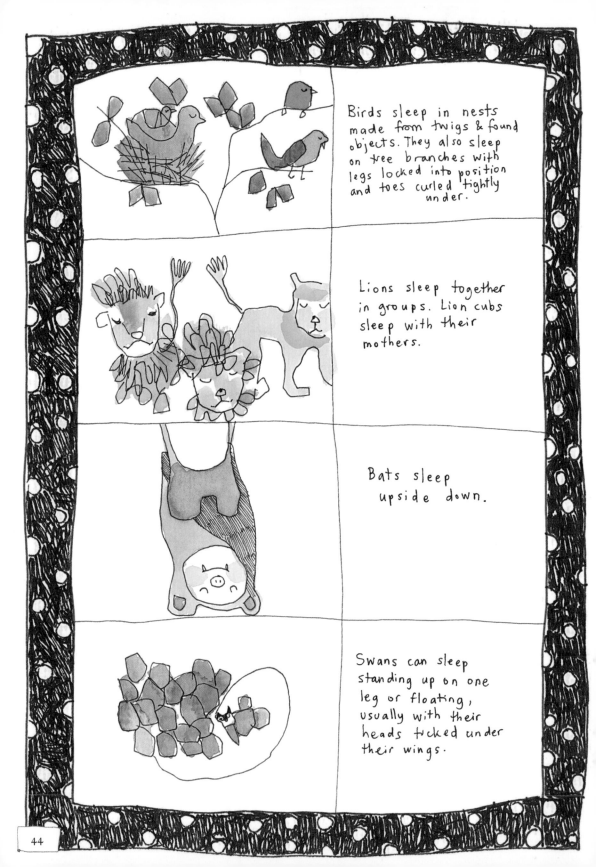

Birds sleep in nests made from twigs & found objects. They also sleep on tree branches with legs locked into position and toes curled tightly under.

Lions sleep together in groups. Lion cubs sleep with their mothers.

Bats sleep upside down.

Swans can sleep standing up on one leg or floating, usually with their heads tucked under their wings.

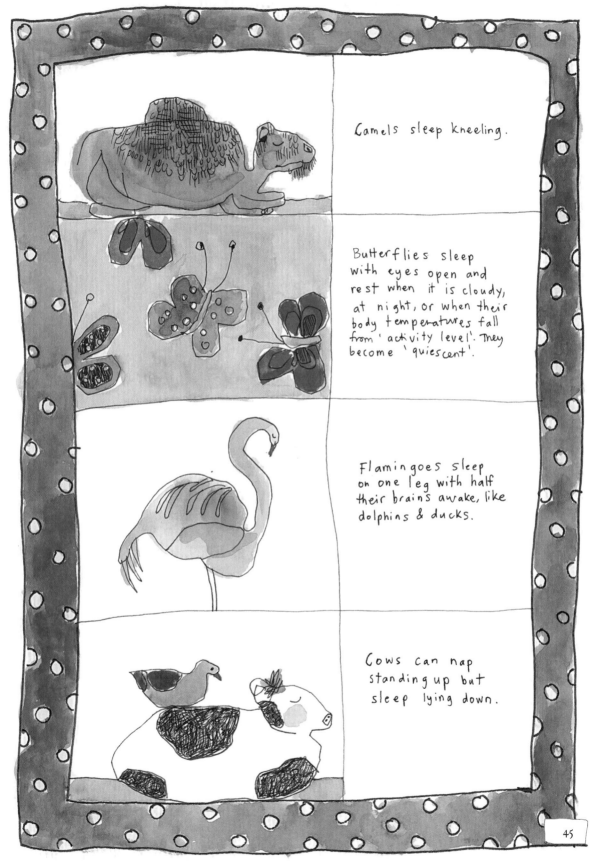

Camels sleep kneeling.

Butterflies sleep
with eyes open and
rest when it is cloudy,
at night, or when their
body temperatures fall
from 'activity level'. They
become 'quiescent'.

Flamingoes sleep
on one leg with half
their brains awake, like
dolphins & ducks.

Cows can nap
standing up but
sleep lying down.

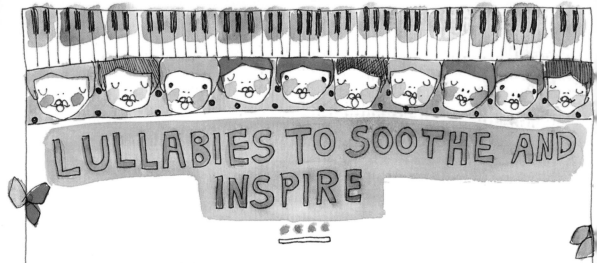

LULLABIES TO SOOTHE AND INSPIRE

LULLABIES HAVE ALWAYS BEEN SUNG BY
PARENTS AROUND THE WORLD TO SOOTHE
AND SETTLE CHILDREN BEFORE SLEEP.

Music alters our heart rate, brainwave patterns and breathing. The simple melodies and repetitiousness of lullabies encourage rest, while the often whimsical, reassuring subject matter promotes sweet dreams. These songs express the tenderness, creativity and faith of the human spirit. Their diversity and beauty is to be celebrated and enjoyed by young and old alike, often allowing a window into another culture.

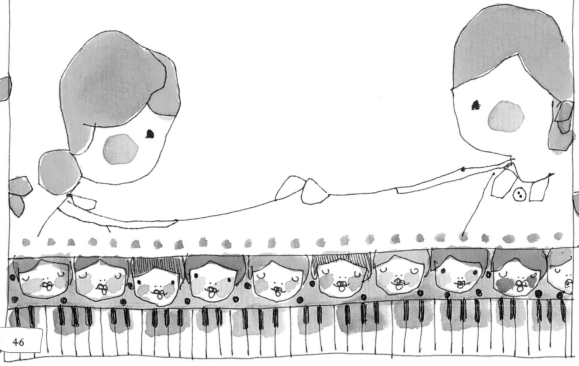

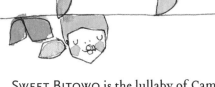

SWEET BITOWO is the lullaby of Cameroonian artist Wes Madiko, who remembers how his mother and grandmother would sing it together to send him to sleep. The lyrics speak of safety and protection, painting a picture of a gentle universe where guardian ancestor spirits watch over, and 'soft stars' soothe and comfort restless children.

HUSH YE, MY BAIRNIE. In Celtic cultures the Suantrai (sleep music) was considered one of music's three main categories (along with the Geantrai (happy songs) and the Goltrai (laments)), expressing themes of maternal love, Mother Nature and angels. 'Hush Ye, My Bairnie' comes from the time when borderland chieftains would lead cattle raids throughout Scotland; the disarmingly simple and beautiful lullabies of the Celtic tradition counter the warlike image of the ancient Celts.

NENNEKO YO. There are a collection of lullabies in Japan that start with 'Nenneko yo', literally 'Sleep, baby child'. The two variations featured here are particularly poignant; the first describes the mother's loving preparation of a special meal for her baby while he sleeps, while in the second example the mother likens her son's rosy cheeks to the colour of the cherry blossom.

FAIS DODO, COLAS, MON PETIT FRÈRE is a charming, traditional French lullaby which soothes and entices with promises of chocolates and sweet cakes, even busy angels above building castles. A night of sweet dreaming would surely follow such lovely thoughts.

MY SLEEP, TAKE IT FROM ME, a very old southern Italian lullaby, transports the sleepy listener to fields of roses where certain blooms must be gathered for particular family members.

THE ELEPHANT'S LULLABY hails from Denmark, and is considered a classic. Written in 1948 by the Danish writer and poet Harald H Lund, its lyrics describe exotic animals in whimsical scenarios, such as zebras putting on striped pyjamas.

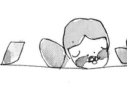

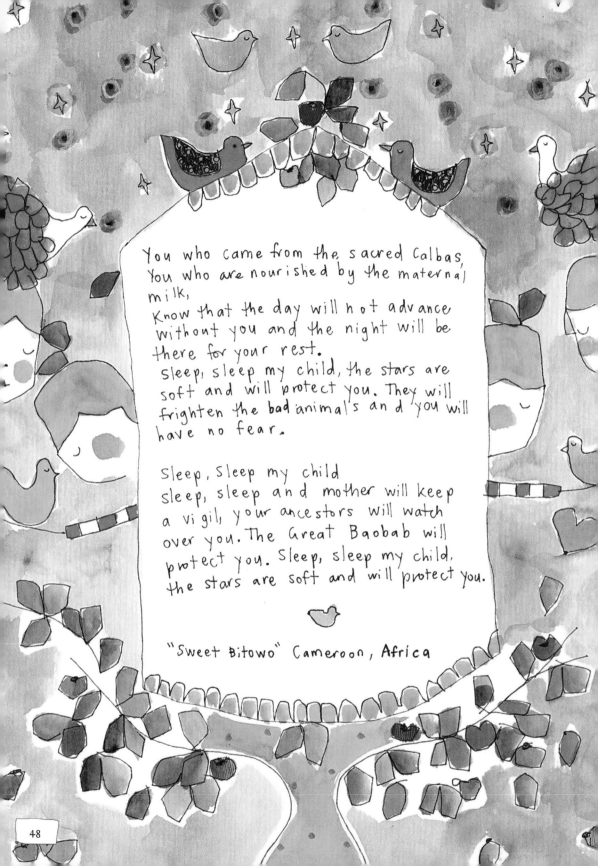

You who came from the sacred Calbas,
You who are nourished by the maternal milk,
Know that the day will not advance
without you and the night will be
there for your rest.
Sleep, sleep my child, the stars are
soft and will protect you. They will
frighten the bad animals and you will
have no fear.

Sleep, Sleep my child
Sleep, sleep and mother will keep
a vigil, your ancestors will watch
over you. The Great Baobab will
protect you. Sleep, sleep my child,
the stars are soft and will protect you.

"Sweet Bitowo" Cameroon, Africa

HUSH YE, MY BAIRNIE

Scotland

Hush ye, my bairnie,
Bonny wee laddie,
When you're a man
You shall follow your daddy
Lift me a coo'n,
a goat and a wether,
Bringing them home
to your mammy together

Hush ye, my bairnie
Bonny wee laddie
Nowt but good things
Ye shall bring to your mammy:
Hare from the mountain
Deer frae the meadow,
Grouse frae the moorland
And trout frae the fountain.

Hush ye, my bairnie
Bonny wee laddie,
Sleep now and close your eyes
Heavy and weary.
Close now your weary eyes,
Rest ye are taking,
Sound be thy sleeping
And bright be thy waking.

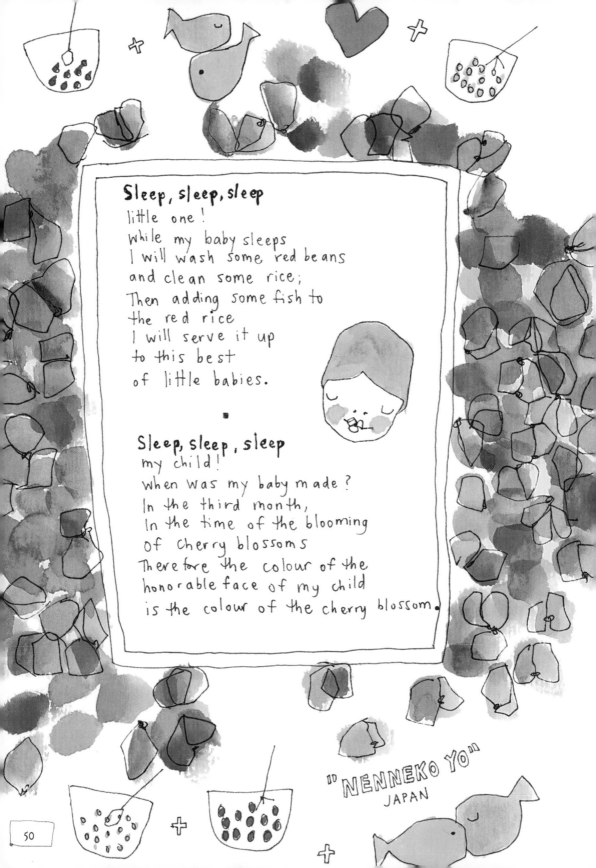

Sleep, sleep, sleep
little one!
while my baby sleeps
I will wash some red beans
and clean some rice;
Then adding some fish to
the red rice
I will serve it up
to this best
of little babies.

Sleep, sleep, sleep
my child!
when was my baby made?
In the third month,
In the time of the blooming
of cherry blossoms
Therefore the colour of the
honorable face of my child
is the colour of the cherry blossom.

"NENNEKO YO"
JAPAN

My sleep, take it from me
and take it to the gardens
and fill its apron
with roses and roses...

The red roses for mother
The red roses for father
and the white roses
for godfather.

"MY SLEEP, TAKE IT FROM ME"
SOUTHERN ITALY.

Now the stars ignite in the blue sky
The half-moon raises its sable
I keep watching, so that the bad mouse
will not sneak into your trunk.
Sleep tight, little jumbo rock-a-bye
Now the wood is getting dark
Now aunty, the old ostrich, is sleeping
And so is your uncle, the rhinoceros.

Now the wild beast calls in its sleep
In the brushwood of the big lianas
And the monkeys sing themselves to sleep
In the cradle of green bananas.
Sleep tight, little jumbo, you little darling
You will want for nothing my friend
tomorrow you will have a coconut
that you will use as a rattle.

A zebra puts on his pyjamas
with black and white stripes
A flying squirrel with fluffy legs
Sits in the dark and squeaks
Sleep tight, little jumbo, you've eaten well?
You know nothing of a mother's worry;
A little plantation with thousands of reeds
That we will pickle tomorrow.

Sleep silently, little jumbo, you little mite
You cute little beetroot!
you asked me to tell you a fairytale
Now you are already sleeping.

EXCERPT FROM 'THE ELEPHANT'S LULLABY'
DENMARK

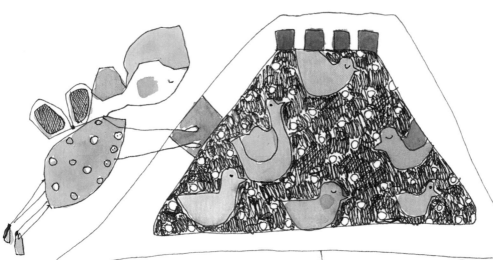

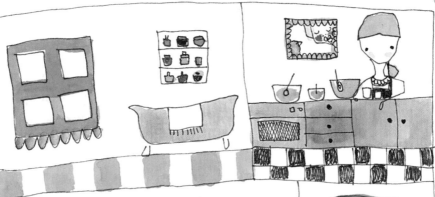

Sleep, my little brother, sleep,
You will have a treat...
Mother is upstairs baking a cake
Papa is downstairs making chocolate
Sleep, my little brother, sleep...
the Angels are above building a castle
for the little brother who is sleeping.
The nice little birds have new songs
for the little brother who is sleeping.
Well sleep, my little brother, sleep,
You will have a treat ...

"Fais Do Do, Colas Mon Petit Frère" FRANCE.

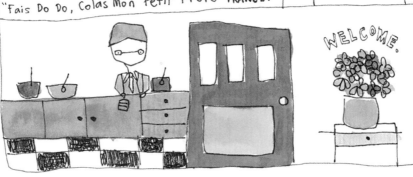

WELCOME.

THE SLEEPY SUPER-MARKET TROLLEY

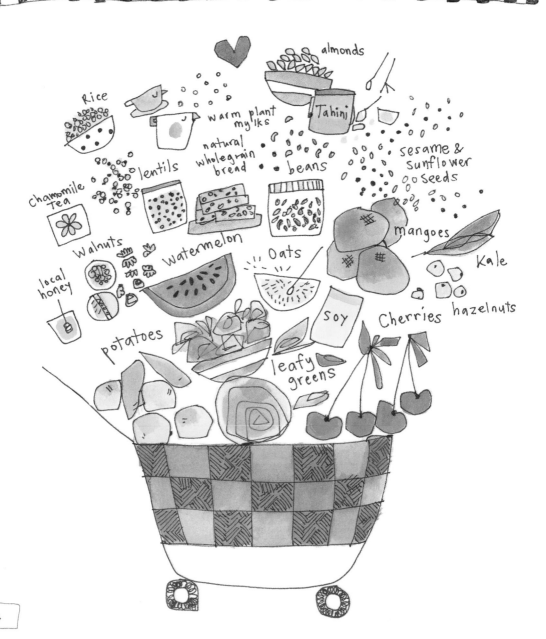

almonds
Rice
warm plant mylks
Tahini
natural wholegrain bread
sesame & sunflower seeds
lentils
beans
chamomile Tea
mangoes
Walnuts
Watermelon
Oats
Kale
local honey
soy
Cherries
hazelnuts
potatoes
leafy greens

THE SLEEPY SUPERMARKET TROLLEY IS STOCKED
TO THE BRIM WITH TRYPTOPHAN-RICH FOOD —
FOOD THAT MAKES US FEEL SLEEPY.

You might be surprised to see hazelnuts, cherries or potatoes in the basket;
indeed, each of these examples contains the naturally occurring amino acid
tryptophan. The body uses tryptophan to make serotonin, a neurotransmitter
that slows down nerve traffic so your brain isn't too busy.

CALCIUM-RICH FOODS such as nuts, seeds and dark leafy greens are considered
'sleepers' as their calcium content aids the tryptophan in producing melatonin. This
reaction manifests itself in those sleepy feelings we sometimes feel after eating. If
used cleverly, certain foods can help us to improve our sleep quality and even counter
insomnia. A glass of warm almond milk before bed could indeed be a very helpful
addition to your tucking-in ritual. A wholegrain sandwich with tahini spread and dark
leafy greens, or a serve of oat porridge with a little sliced mango or some cherries will
also bring on that siesta feeling!

LIGHT MEALS AT NIGHT are highly recommended for everybody, especially those
seeking to enhance the quality of their slumber. Large meals with a high fat content,
highly seasoned or spicy meals, even too much garlic, tend to interfere with sleep.

A LACK OF SLEEP or disrupted sleep can lead to impaired mood, memory
and concentration, a dampening of the immune system and a compromised sense
of coordination. Eating too late will also affect your sleep quality. An early evening meal
will allow your body time to digest your food effectively and allow you
to feel more comfortable when you lie down. Remembering to exercise regularly,
even taking a little walk after dinner before you tuck in to bed,
will aid digestion and encourage replenishing slumber.

THE MIDNIGHT SNACK...

BELOW YOU WILL FIND A FEW MEALS CONCOCTED FROM
INGREDIENTS IN THE SLEEPY SUPERMARKET TROLLEY.
THESE LITTLE MEALS ARE BOUND TO BRING ON THE
YAWNING AND LEAVE YOU SNOOZING BLISSFULLY.

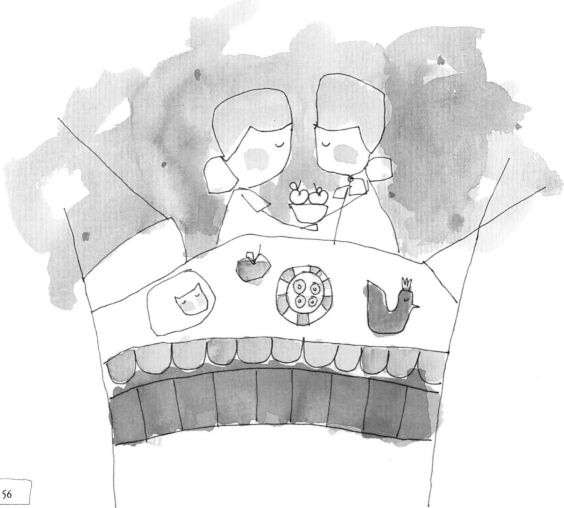

GETTING SLEEEEPY ?...

Almond butter on toast

A little bowl of coconut yogurt with cherries

Warm lentil and vegetable soup

Rice cakes with hummus and leafy greens

Baked potato with green salad

A handful of walnuts

A slice or two of fresh watermelon

Warm nut or soy milk with a pinch of vanilla
and a little honey

Oat porridge with coconut milk and hazelnuts

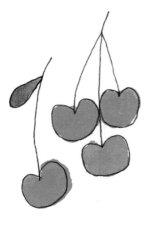

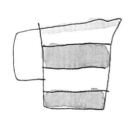

NB: While under the umbrella of the 'midnight snack', some of the more substantial examples in this list are more appropriate for evening meals, eaten a good few hours before tucking in.

Look to the Sleepy Supermarket Trolley on pages 54–55 for a pinch of inspiration and invent your own sleepy snacks to ensure a spectacular snooze.

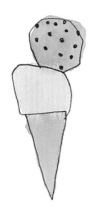

PYJAMA PARTY TIME!

YOU MIGHT BE TUCKED IN BED FEELING WEARY, UNWELL OR
UNINSPIRED, OR YOU MIGHT SIMPLY BE AN ENTHUSIASTIC
LOVER OF ALL THINGS BED.

Sometimes calling a pyjama party is the best medicine. If you're not well
enough or simply unwilling to emerge from your cosy kingdom, simply ask those
you love to bring the party to you! For an added sense of cosiness and to match
your mood, the dress code should be anything bed-worthy – flannelette jarmies,
ugg boots, bed socks, sleeping caps and snuggly dressing gowns.

You might encourage your guests to bring along some edible delights,
or whip up some of your own homemade comfort food to share (see Comfort
Food Recipes, pages 86–93). For beverages you might make a generous pot
of ginger tea, or hot chocolate with melting marshmallows. Grabbing a DVD
and dimming the lights can provide great entertainment – just ensure
it's something light-hearted that everyone can enjoy.

Good old-fashioned board games may also be incorporated into the festivities,
or if you're mobile a little piñata or 'Pin the tail on the donkey' always go
down a treat. A readymade invitation to distribute amongst your posse is on
the opposite page; all you will need to do is fill in the gaps and locate your best
pyjamas. Just because you're tucked in doesn't mean you can't celebrate.
On the contrary, make it an occasion to snuggle back and party on!

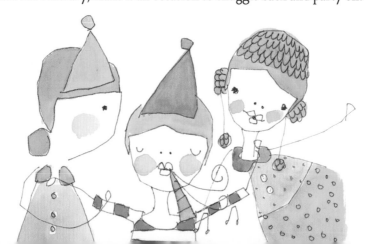

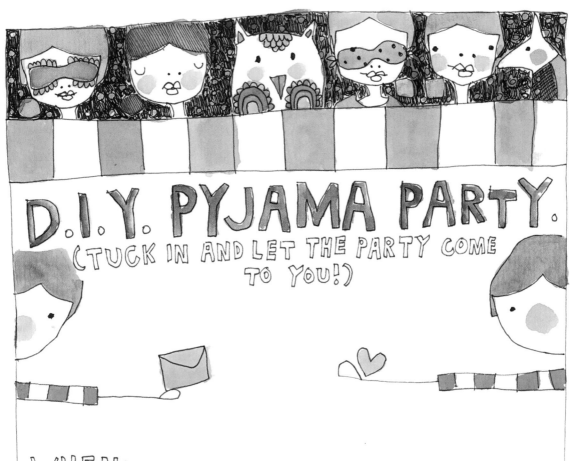

D.I.Y. PYJAMA PARTY.
(TUCK IN AND LET THE PARTY COME TO YOU!)

WHEN:

WHERE:

DRESS CODE:

RSVP:

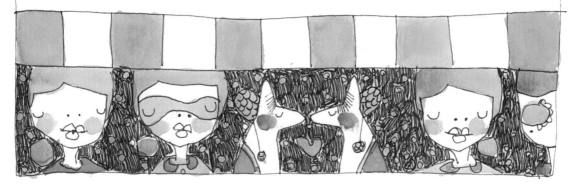

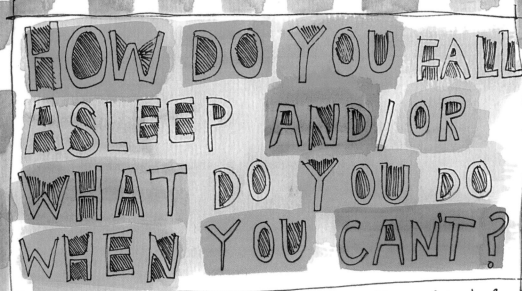

HOW DO YOU FALL ASLEEP AND/OR WHAT DO YOU DO WHEN YOU CAN'T?

In search of precious sleeping tips, I asked family, friends & strangers from around the world for their unique night-owl secrets! Here are their unusual and inspiring answers:

WHO?	ABOUT:	SECRET ANSWER:
CARM-ELLA	Collector, Shop keeper and Wise owl MELBOURNE	Fluffs her pillows, makes a warm cup of tea and snuggles back in with a book.
BOB H	Art Director SYDNEY	Swims imaginary laps of his local pool.
KYLIE W	Podiatrist and super chef BOTANY	Gets up and puts all her worrying thoughts on paper to clear her mind.
SARAH G	Ceramic Artist and social worker DULWICH HILL	Enjoys a warm bath or practises her headstands.
BELA H	Lawyer and party maker BERLIN	Solves all the world's problems or wonders what he would do if he won the lottery.
TRENT	Nurse and science student TASMANIA	Likes to read or record thoughts on paper. When desperate Trent meditates and performs a series of stretches.

JENNY P	Green Thumb AVALON	Drinks chamomile tea and listens to late-night radio.
RUSSIAN LUCY	Linguist ROMA/ITALIA	Invents her own fanciful bedtime stories and failing that - makes a warm cup of tea and plays them over in black & white
JULIE S	Fashionista with best laugh SYDNEY	Turns the lights out and closes her eyes, imagining that she is floating above her bed seeing the image of herself sleeping soundly. Julie believes that the powers of visualisation work every time!
ELIZABETH B	Artist and Letter Writer MELBOURNE	Loves it when someone dear to her gently strokes her forehead. It was her mother's way of soothing her as a baby.
JAKE FROM LONDON	Pianist and Academic MET IN KAS, TURKEY	Makes origami.
BENNI K	Windmill Maker KREUZBERG, BERLIN	Reads a book in bed with a warm cup of milk & honey, or a little glass of wine.
MADI S	Traveller, Anthropologist Musical talent THE WORLD	Plays with her memories and builds life-sized models of the future.
BENNI BASH	Pilot, Psychologist Nurse, Painter LANCASHIRE, ENGLAND	Calculates the square root of integers until the numbers are so big that she can't keep track of them.
JACQUIE H	Teacher, Serious Ukulele talent DARWIN	Tenses all body muscles for twenty seconds - then relaxes. Repeats three times.
TASHI -LA	Writer, gatherer, artist TASMANIA	Focusing on the feeling of her breath going in and out stills her mind - or reading until she's sleepy.
BRONWYN B C	Performance Artist MELBOURNE	Tells herself stories that turn into visual journeys that turn into dreams...
LIA & RAF	Academics & Socialites FRIULI, ITALIA	Dream up new combinations for home made gelato.

	NORA J	Grandma Extraordinaire SYDNEY	Walks about her house, counting her steps. Says the rosary.
	MONICA T	Singer, writer performer, chef SYDNEY	Does some knitting, or watches old black and white movies while nibbling on cookies.
	KAT H	Gallery owner & Agent SYDNEY	Remembers the wonderful sounds, tastes and smells of Christmas Days spent together with her family and cousins at her Grandma's house.
	MR LINDEMANN	P.R, Ice skater, Graffiti Artist & more BERLIN	Longs for his faraway love.
	LUCY H	Film Maker STANMORE SYDNEY	Listens to stories on cassette tapes (special love: Rudyard Kipling's 'Just so stories')
	JESS F	Designer & Photographer AUSTRIA	Reads Moby Dick.
	NIKKO G	Traveller, Poet, Business man, Brother (currently in Morocco)	Listens to talkback radio.
	TIMO	DJ, Event Co-ordinator Party Specialist BERLIN	Goes out dancing.
	ED	Banker and Business man SYDNEY	Reflects on the highlights of his day or composes intricate pieces of imaginary music.
	HANNAH M	Social worker, musician & photographer SYDNEY	Reads stories out loud to her partner until they are both asleep.
	FIONA L	Lawyer, Gallery owner & night owl SYDNEY	Cuddles her little boy Owen while he sleeps, becoming sleepy & calm.
	RON G	Interior Designer POTTS POINT, BUNDANOON	Drinks cups of tea on his rooftop, listens to talkback radio and doesn't worry about his sleeplessness. Ron is a consumate night owl.

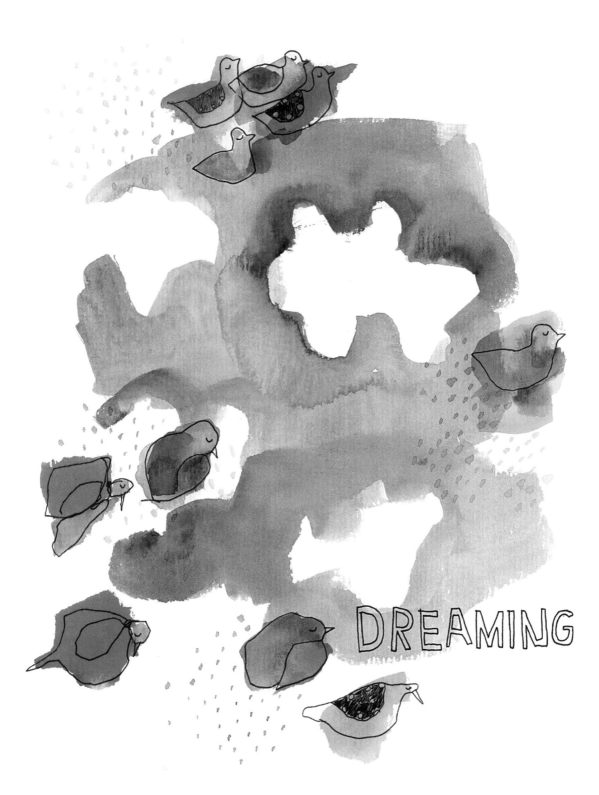

THE SECRET STORIES BEHIND OUR DREAMS

PEOPLE HAVE LONG BEEN FASCINATED BY THE MEANING
OF DREAMS, AND THE MYSTERY OF THE DREAMING EXPERIENCE. THE
MESSAGES OUR DREAMS BRING TO US CAN BE HEALING, INSPIRING AND
DEEPLY INSIGHTFUL.

ANCIENT EGYPTIANS RECORDED their dreams in hieroglyphics, as well as theories on dream symbolism. The Egyptian *Chester Beatty Papyri* are some of the most ancient texts on dreaming known to humanity.

People who dreamed especially vivid dreams were considered to be blessed, while those who interpreted dreams were seen as almost divine. Priests were consulted to interpret dreams, as they were perceived to contain vital messages from the gods. The practice of 'dream incubation' began in ancient Egypt, whereby the ill or troubled individual would sleep in a temple and then report the night's dreams directly to a priest.

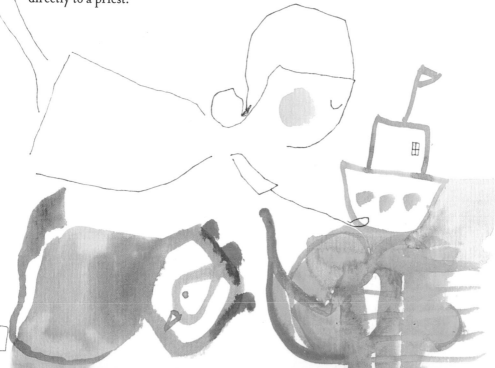

In Ancient Greece, dreams were also interpreted by priests and used as part of the healing process. Ill people were directed to temples where the 'gods of the body' had their shrines. After performing religious ceremonies they slept, hoping to have the dream that would renew their health. The Roman philosopher Heraclitus, who wrote the first comprehensive book on dreams (*The Oneirocriticon*), was first to suggest that dreams were the creations of the mind. Such ideas would later be explored by modern thinkers such as Freud and Jung. Freud theorised that dreams expressed hidden desires, while Jung saw them as messages from ourselves.

In Native American culture ancestors are believed to live in dreams in the forms of flora and fauna. Dreaming links the dreamer with their past and their spirit ancestors. Indigenous Australians use the term 'The Dreaming' or 'Dreamtime' to encapsulate the past, the present and the future. Dreaming stories tell of the creation of the world, and explain why animals, places and things look and feel the way they do. They are passed down and brought alive through ritual, art, spoken word and dance.

Chinese thinkers proposed that the soul and spirit left the body during dreaming, going to an actual place to 'visit' for the night. They feared that if suddenly woken their souls would fail to return to their bodies and would float, eternally displaced. The Chinese practised 'dream incubation', seeking not only healing and enlightenment, but inspiration for paintings and music.

The following pages explore the most common dream symbols and offer ideas for their interpretation. The significance of your dreams, however, will be particular and special to you. Bringing along your own experiences, history and ideas to these analyses will be essential to discovering some of the hidden treasures in your private whimsical world.

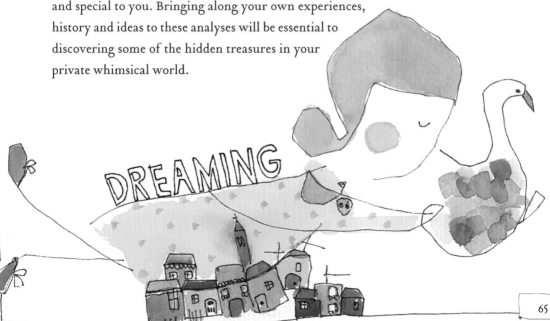

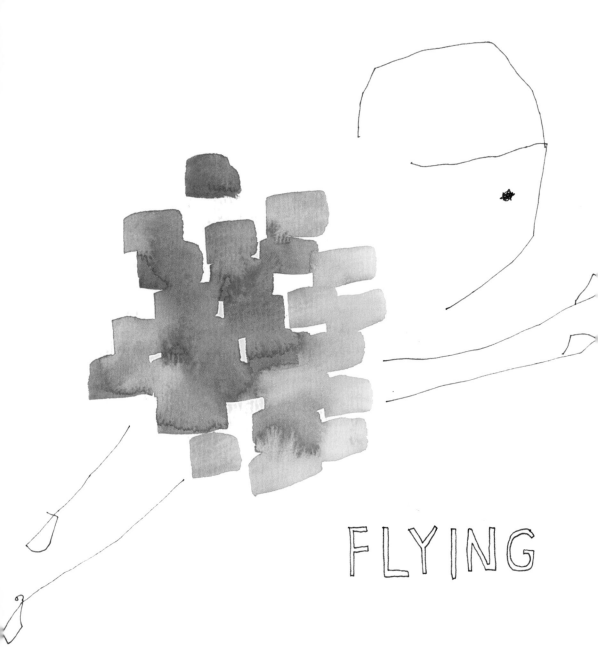

FLYING

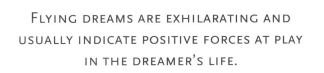

FLYING DREAMS ARE EXHILARATING AND
USUALLY INDICATE POSITIVE FORCES AT PLAY
IN THE DREAMER'S LIFE.

Flying high over pleasant scenery represents being 'on top' of a situation, finding a solution, or learning a valuable lesson. Feeling in control of your flight path indicates your sense of power and ability. If you feel free and comfortable when sky-high, performing acrobatics and using your arms and feet for direction, you can be assured that life is good. Be proud and excited about the fruits of your labour! If you feel uncomfortable, you might be overly ambitious or fear challenges or success. Flying over muddy water warns you to keep your private affairs close as others are watching and may not have the best intentions.

OUR ANCESTORS associated flying dreams with fleeing from struggle. Today, they are still associated with mental recovery, or being liberated. Flying low to the ground suggests sickness or uneasy states from which the dreamer will recover, while flying over green trees foretells that you will suffer temporary embarrassment but will have a flood of prosperity.

If you experience the wonderfully giddy feelings of lightness, openness and freedom, you are being asked to carry these feelings with you in your waking life. You move more lightly and realise you may overcome the forces that ground you.

Do you find powerlines, mountains or trees blocking your flight path? These obstructions represent actual obstacles or frustrations in your waking life that stop you from achieving your goals. They may also represent a lack of self-confidence. A particularly powerful version of such a dream message is when you fail to take off at all. Look at your life circumstances and seek to discover what is holding you back.

OPEN
SEA

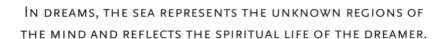

IN DREAMS, THE SEA REPRESENTS THE UNKNOWN REGIONS OF THE MIND AND REFLECTS THE SPIRITUAL LIFE OF THE DREAMER.

The way in which water is dreamt about is also said to be significant: seeing an artificial lagoon, canal or swimming pool suggests that your spiritual flow is being obstructed by conventional ideals, while dreaming of a boundless, open sea indicates the abundance and freedom of your spirituality. Dreaming of the sea may show that you are now ready to explore the intuitive and instinctive facets of yourself – your creativity. Jumping into water signifies a request for you to 'get into life'. To see a sailor in your dreams indicates a desire for adventure, freedom and excitement. What do you yearn to do? Where do you wish to go? Seeing a sailboat in your dreams symbolises your emotional self and how you navigate through various situations in your life. Is your ocean tumultuous and rocky? Is it smooth, peaceful and quiet? Or is the wind shifting, suggesting you need to adapt to a new situation?

ACCORDING TO GUSTAVUS HINDMAN MILLER in his epic *10 000 Dreams Interpreted*, hearing the sea sigh in a dream foretells that you will be fated to a life of solitude, fruitlessness and weariness. On the other hand, for a young woman to dream that she glides swiftly over the sea with her lover foretells an exchange of vows and a life coloured by hope, promise and joy. Consider the imagery in your sea dream: the nature of the water, and your emotions toward entering or traversing it. It is most likely your dream encapsulates the way you are handling a particular emotional journey in your waking life, drawing attention to your feelings of readiness or excitement, capability or fear. Sea dreams highlight the power of our human instinct and intuition; they remind us that our thoughts and feelings shape our worlds.

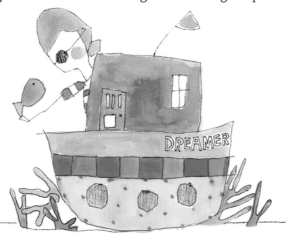

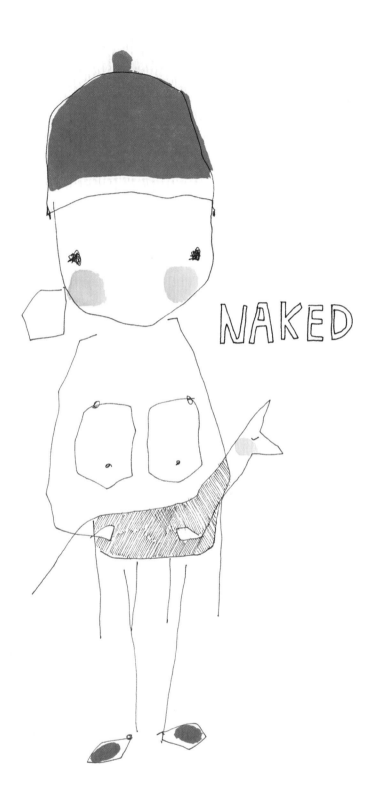

NAKED

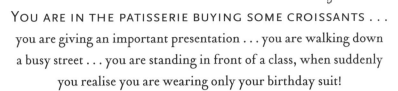

YOU ARE IN THE PATISSERIE BUYING SOME CROISSANTS . . .
you are giving an important presentation . . . you are walking down
a busy street . . . you are standing in front of a class, when suddenly
you realise you are wearing only your birthday suit!

SUCH DREAMS ARE common and can symbolise various things, depending on their context and timing. Feeling mortified about your nudity in such a dream indicates shame, guilt, or a sense of inferiority. Clothes are forms of concealment and have the power to hide or change your identity. To feel exposed and defenceless in a naked dream denotes a fear of being ridiculed and disgraced. Such dreams often occur around times of exposure, or when you are seeking to impress, such as during an interview, presentation, or a new relationship.

Naked dreams may indicate your fear of failure, or of revealing your true self. Dreams about nakedness may also indicate a longing for a return to the innocence of childhood; to the real you, stripped of pretence and social conditioning. During stressful periods, such dreams may represent the wish to abandon adult responsibilities and run free.

DREAMS IN WHICH you are disgusted by other people's nudity suggest your fear of discovering your own or someone else's possibly ugly side, their 'naked truth'. On the contrary, accepting and appreciating others' nudity suggests your ability to respect and recognise others for who they are. Dreams in which you are happy and carefree in your nakedness indicate a sense of healthy self-love and pride, as well as honesty and openness.

Another message from your naked dream may be that while you seek to be noticed, you go about it the wrong way. Is your dream asking you to look in the mirror and allow yourself to just be? If no-one else notices your nudity, is it a call for you to look at your own fears about yourself? Are they ungrounded? While mothers used to warn daughters that naked dreams signified the imminent exposure of scandal, gypsies believed that good fortune awaited the person who dreamed of being naked, especially if the dream was lit by the stars.

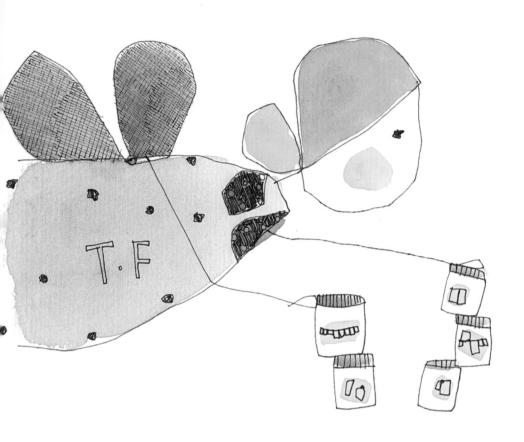

TEETH

IKE US MODERN DREAMERS, those of yesteryear sought interpretation and guidance after troubling teeth dreams: crumbling teeth, teeth falling out with just a little tap, growing crooked or even rotting. Such dreams tend to leave lasting, often disturbing images in our minds. Funnily enough, other characters in such dreams do not seem to notice or care about the ugly, missing or loose teeth; they are only a concern to the dreamer. Some dreamers imagine looking in mirrors before important meetings or social situations, only to notice that some of their teeth are missing. Such a dream commonly invokes shock, panic or disgust. One theory is that teeth dreams represent anxiety about physical appearance. Are you overly concerned about how others perceive you? Do you fear embarrassment to do with your body?

IN A WORLD WHERE all too often judgements are cast on superficial grounds, such anxiety is tragically common. These dreams might signal an opportunity to show yourself some love and appreciation, and to focus not on what you lack but on what you have to give.

Another explanation for teeth dreams is concerned with power. We use teeth to bite, chew, gnaw and tear. Their loss can signify powerlessness, inferiority or a lack of self-confidence. Tooth loss occurs at two distinct stages of life, first in childhood with the loss of milk teeth, and later in old age. At the first stage, children are often taking on new responsibilities and experiencing a rite of passage into a more grown-up reality. Such change is accompanied by a sense of thrill and excitement, but also with fear of the new, the larger world and the unknown. At the second stage, the loss or decay of teeth can accompany a fear of waning and loss of control. In Greek culture dreaming of teeth signifies that a family member or close friend is very sick, or even close to death.

Teeth are useful when they are inside our mouths, but when they fall out they lose their function. Some analysts have likened 'teeth-falling-out dreams' to a feeling of being unheard. While the dreamer's words are important in their mouth, they become worthless when converted into speech. Accordingly, some theorists suggest that teeth dreams indicate you are having a hard time being heard or acknowledged. Do you feel your thoughts, feelings and opinions are not valued or heard? Perhaps your teeth dreams are asking you to look at your relationships and aim to find your voice, a new way to express yourself and to ensure that you are heard.

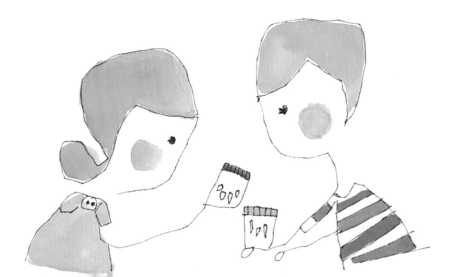

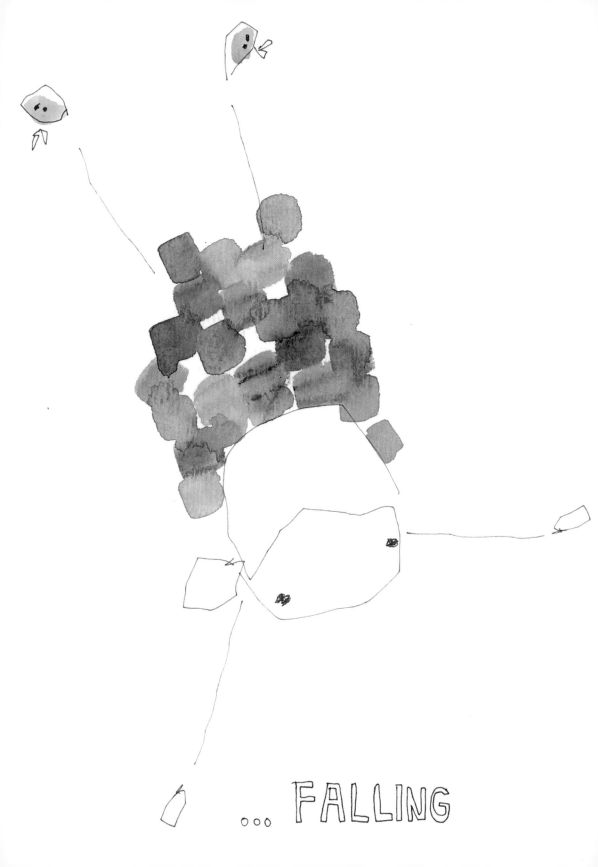

... FALLING

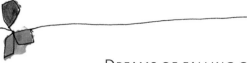

DREAMS OF FALLING OFTEN HAPPEN DURING THE
VERY FIRST STAGES OF SLEEP, AND ARE ACCOMPANIED BY
A PHYSICAL SENSATION OF ACTUALLY FALLING.

This muscle spasm felt in the arms and legs, or the whole body, otherwise known as a 'hypnagogic myoclonic twitch', can be the result of a drop in blood pressure or even the movement of fluid in the middle ear. The jerking action often makes the sleeper wake up and become quickly alert and responsive to possible environmental threats. Research has found that when astronauts are in space they dream that everything floats! Some say that falling in dreams is simply a physical sensation rather than anything deeper or symbolic, and that something as simple as having a harder bed will minimise the frequency of 'sleep falling'. Evolutionists have linked falling in dreams to times long past when remaining high in trees as necessary for our survival. Others see falling dreams as indicative of insecurities, instabilities or anxieties in our waking lives.

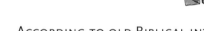

ACCORDING TO OLD BIBLICAL INTERPRETATIONS, dreams about falling indicated that the dreamer was on an ungodly path. They indicated a fall from grace, poor decision making, or shameful behaviour. Seeing and experiencing ourselves gradually falling in our dreams may indicate a need for us to comfort ourselves in connection to a poor decision we have made. The act of falling also involves letting go. Other interpretations suggest that the dreamer may fear the loss of someone or something important to them. As falling is something that usually happens to us rather than something we wish to experience, such dreams ask us to look at circumstances in our waking lives that may be unfavourable, but that are out of our control. The feeling of falling comes with a sense of loss of control. In which parts of your life do you feel you have lost grip? Are you feeling overwhelmed or unsupported? Or is your dream foretelling a fall? Perhaps you are acting in a high-handed fashion that is disproportionate to your real capabilities? Consider the timing and context of your falling dream. Seek correlations in your waking life that may be responsible for your angst, and take positive action to stay on your feet. Last but not least, check your house for a broken step, a loose handrail or a wobbly chair. In your subconscious you may have intuited an accident waiting to happen!

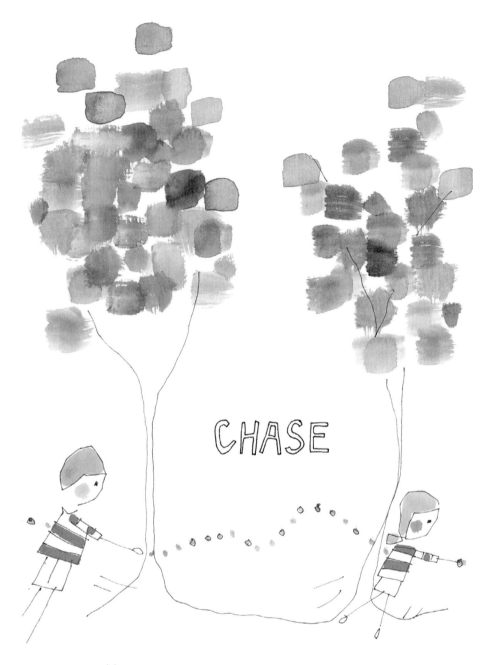

CHASE

HAVE YOU EVER WOKEN FROM A DISTURBING DREAM
OF BEING CHASED, RELIEVED TO REALISE YOU ARE SAFE,
SNUGGLED BETWEEN THE SHEETS?

Chase dreams feel very real, leaving a lasting impression on the dreamer. They are often recurrent, and trigger memories of childhood vulnerability. Looking at the nature of the chase helps in decoding the meaning of your particular dream.

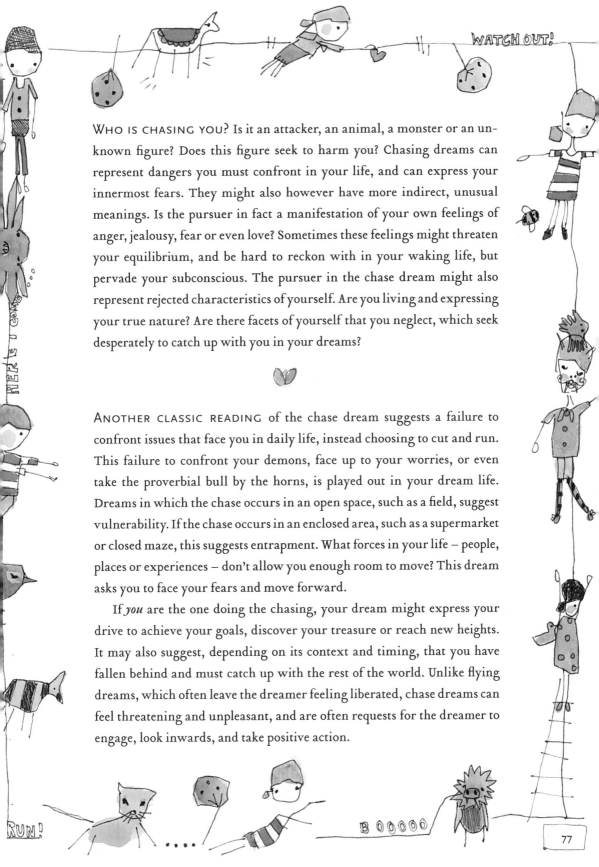

WHO IS CHASING YOU? Is it an attacker, an animal, a monster or an unknown figure? Does this figure seek to harm you? Chasing dreams can represent dangers you must confront in your life, and can express your innermost fears. They might also however have more indirect, unusual meanings. Is the pursuer in fact a manifestation of your own feelings of anger, jealousy, fear or even love? Sometimes these feelings might threaten your equilibrium, and be hard to reckon with in your waking life, but pervade your subconscious. The pursuer in the chase dream might also represent rejected characteristics of yourself. Are you living and expressing your true nature? Are there facets of yourself that you neglect, which seek desperately to catch up with you in your dreams?

ANOTHER CLASSIC READING of the chase dream suggests a failure to confront issues that face you in daily life, instead choosing to cut and run. This failure to confront your demons, face up to your worries, or even take the proverbial bull by the horns, is played out in your dream life. Dreams in which the chase occurs in an open space, such as a field, suggest vulnerability. If the chase occurs in an enclosed area, such as a supermarket or closed maze, this suggests entrapment. What forces in your life – people, places or experiences – don't allow you enough room to move? This dream asks you to face your fears and move forward.

If *you* are the one doing the chasing, your dream might express your drive to achieve your goals, discover your treasure or reach new heights. It may also suggest, depending on its context and timing, that you have fallen behind and must catch up with the rest of the world. Unlike flying dreams, which often leave the dreamer feeling liberated, chase dreams can feel threatening and unpleasant, and are often requests for the dreamer to engage, look inwards, and take positive action.

DREAM CATCHER

ORIGINATING FROM NATIVE AMERICAN INDIAN CULTURE AND TRADITION, DREAM CATCHERS WERE ORIGINALLY CRAFTED FROM A WILLOW HOOP THROUGH WHICH VARIOUS MATERIALS OF SACRED AND PERSONAL MEANING WERE BOUND TOGETHER IN A WEB OF THREADS.

OBJECTS SUCH AS feathers, stones, beads and charms were gathered for artistic use. The idea of hanging a dream catcher near a sleeping place was to filter dreams through its web, only allowing good dreams to reach the sleeper; bad or haunting dreams would be caught up in the web, only to dissolve in the pure morning light. Some say that from a jumble of dreams, or rather a mixture of good and bad spirits in the night air, only the good could enter through a hole in the centre of the web, gliding down the feathers to the tucked-in dreamer.

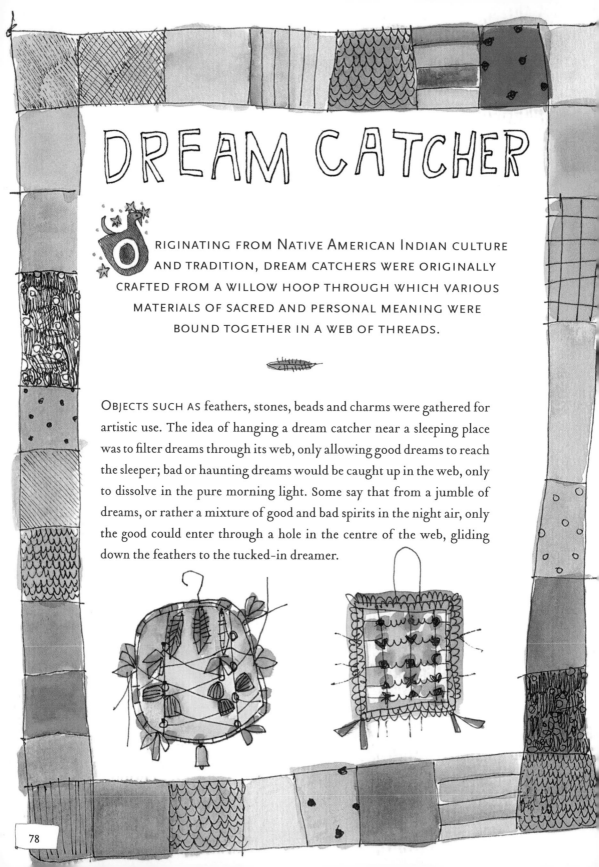

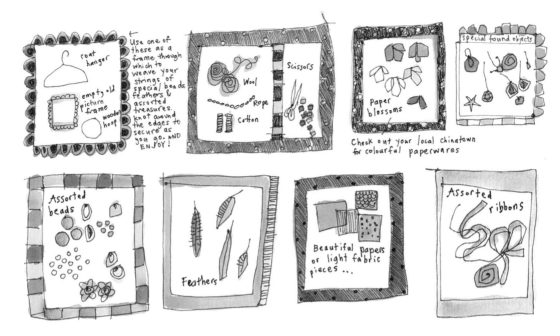

Use one of these as a frame, through which to weave your strings of special/beads, feathers & assorted treasures. Knot around the edges to secure as you go. AND ENJOY!

coat hanger

empty old picture frame

wooden hoop

Wool

Rope

Cotton

Scissors

Paper blossoms

special found objects

Check out your local Chinatown for colourful paperwares

Assorted beads

Feathers

Beautiful papers or light fabric pieces ...

Assorted ribbons

THE BIODEGRADABLE ASPECT of the natural materials used by traditional crafts-people also held a special meaning. By the time a child was old enough to negotiate the various night spirits at play, the leaves and natural objects in their dream catcher would be naturally decomposing, marking a rite of passage; an entry into adulthood. The significance of the hoop shape, the circle, is also central to Native American Indian philosophy. It was seen to represent unity and strength.

TODAY, DREAM CATCHERS have travelled far and wide from their origin. To the dismay of native craftspeople, dream catchers as physical objects have become highly commercialised and somewhat exploited abroad, displaced from their sacred context and meaning.

However, if created mindfully and with respect, using objects that hold a special meaning for you, the true essence of the dream catcher can be celebrated and reborn. Your dream catcher can be symbolic of your own beliefs and history, woven with beautiful, meaningful objects that provide nightly positive reinforcement, and a focus for reflecting upon the mysterious wonders of dreaming.

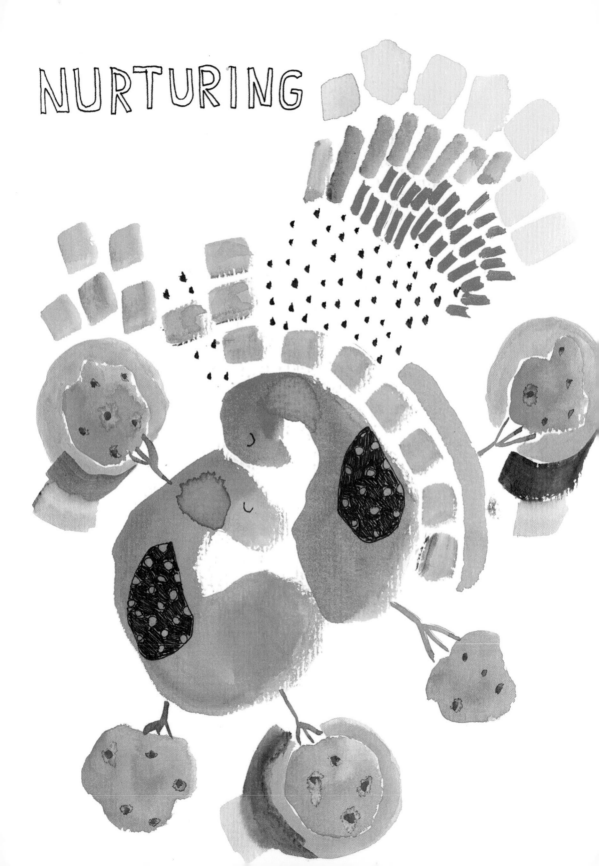

NURTURING

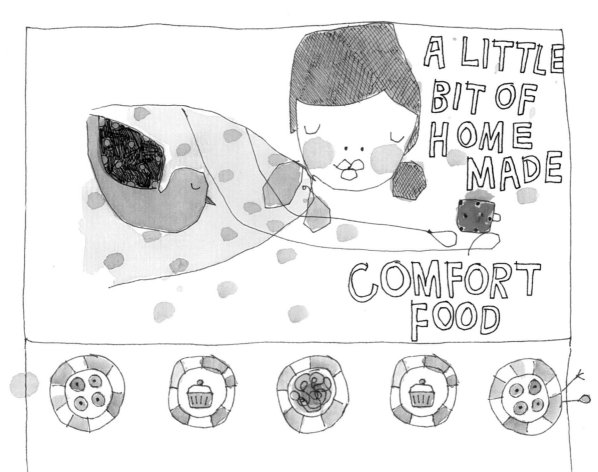

A LITTLE BIT OF HOME MADE

COMFORT FOOD

IT IS NO SECRET THAT FOOD CAN BE A WAY TO THE HEART.
HEART-WARMING, COMFORTING FOOD MADE WITH LOVE
AND CARE CAN BE A MARVELLOUS HEALING AGENT.

Nourishing foods can help our bodies to recover from illness and lift
our spirits. It is a lovely gesture to prepare comfort food for somebody who is
unwell, and naturally it is a wonderful thing to be on the receiving end of such
an offering. The following recipes have been selected because their warmth
and goodness are conducive to healing and recovery. They are also foods
appropriate for a pinch of 'tucked-in dining' on those bed-bound days.
May they bring joy and comfort to you and those you love.

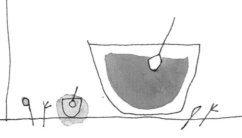

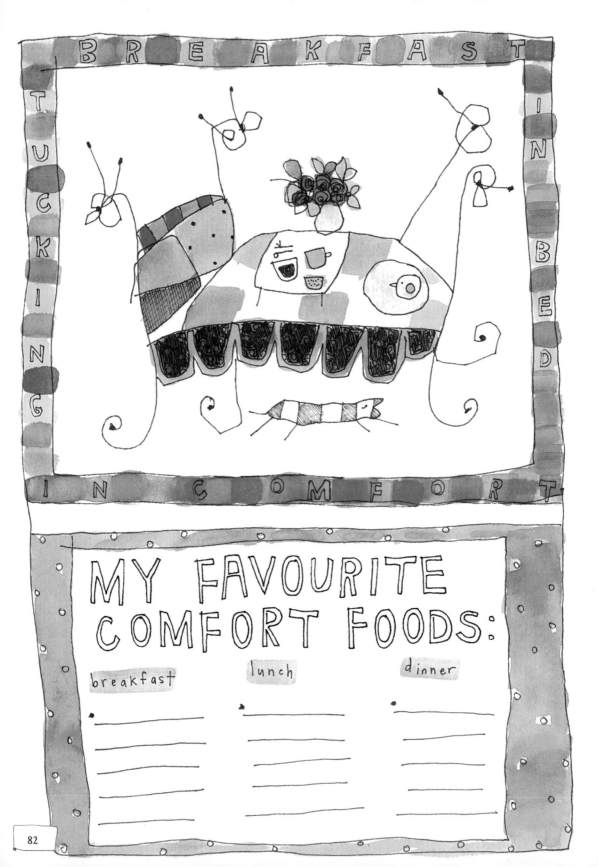

DINING IN

When you're tucked in bed warm and snug, but have worked up quite an appetite getting creative with your shadow puppets, designing your dream catcher and writing haiku poetry (see pp 102-103), it might be time to ring your little bell for room service. Some of us might be lucky enough to have a dedicated friend, loved one, or very well-trained pet to bring various nibbles and supplies to our bedsides. In the event such helping hands are unavailable it is also possible to set your own tea tray and return with it to the comfort of snuggledom.

Food is like edible love. Food prepared with passion, awareness and loving feelings aids recovery from illness, strengthens the body and warms the heart. Have you ever noticed how much more wonderful a cup of tea tastes when made for you by a loved one and hand delivered? Or how much nicer your own homemade biscuits, warm from the oven, taste than supermarket varieties?!

When tucked in, comfort foods become particularly important. Try "Pumpkin soup for the soul" (see recipe on pp 88-89), a pot of fresh ginger tea or a little bit of honey on toast. Treat yourself.

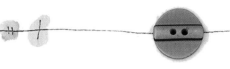
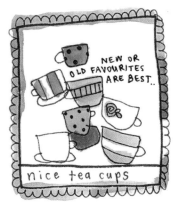

NEW OR OLD FAVOURITES ARE BEST..

nice tea cups

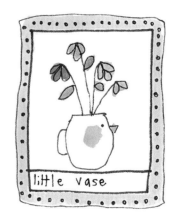

little vase

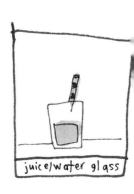

juice/water glass

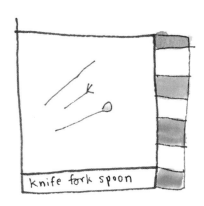

knife fork spoon

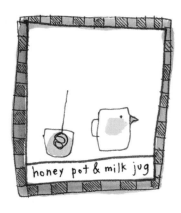

honey pot & milk jug

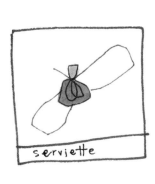

serviette

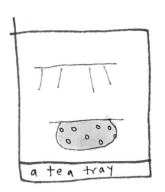

a tea tray

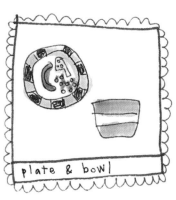

plate & bowl

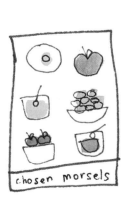

chosen morsels

PREPARING A TEA TRAY

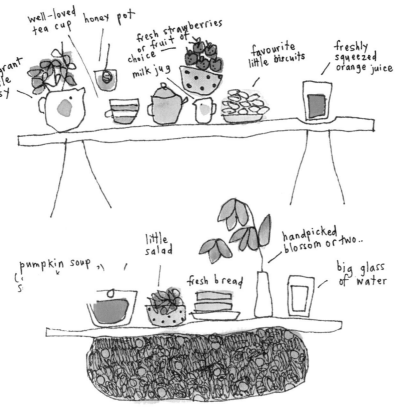

fragrant little posy

well-loved tea cup

honey pot

fresh strawberries or fruit of choice

milk jug

favourite little biscuits

freshly squeezed orange juice

pumpkin soup

little salad

fresh bread

handpicked blossom or two..

big glass of water

Tea trays can be found in all different sizes and boasting different appealing features. You may desire the practical addition of a cup holder, nifty pop-out legs or built-in crockery. Or you may prefer the variety that cleverly sits atop a cushion and easily finds itself a cosy and convenient spot. These diagrams show both a sweet & savoury style tea tray, with suggestions of delicious morsels to nurture, strengthen and fill. Don't forget the flowers: their freshness and beauty brings a breath of spring into bed!

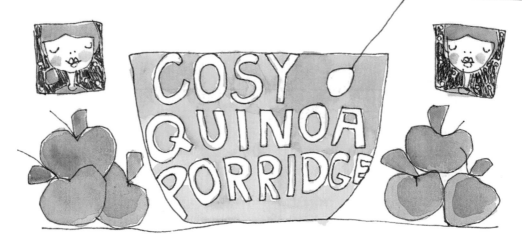

COSY QUINOA PORRIDGE

This comforting and nutritious porridge draws on the power of quinoa, a grain cultivated in the Andes since at least 3000 BC. The ancient Incas referred to quinoa as 'The Mother Grain'. Not only does quinoa boast lots of protein, iron and calcium, it contains essential amino acids as well as valuable B and E vitamins.

6 dried Turkish figs, quartered
4 fresh apricots, quartered
1½ tablespoons sultanas
juice of 1 orange

1 cup (170g) quinoa
2 tablespoons coconut yogurt (optional)
pistachios or dry-roasted almonds
    and maple syrup (optional), to serve

Place Turkish figs, apricots and sultanas in a saucepan. Add orange juice and a little water (enough to just cover the fruit). Cover and bring to the boil then reduce heat to low and allow fruit to simmer until it is the consistency of a compote (15–20 minutes).

Meanwhile, add 2 cups of water to the quinoa, cover and bring to the boil over a medium heat. Turn the flame to low and allow to simmer gently for 12–15 minutes.

Once most of the water has been absorbed, remove from heat and allow to stand for about 3 minutes.

Fluff the cooked quinoa lightly with a fork, then place portions in the centre of your chosen bowls. Serve with generous dollops of fruit compote and coconut yogurt. Top with pistachio nuts or dry-roasted almonds, and a little swirl of maple syrup if desired.

For a sweeter, stickier and creamier dish, or as a substitute for yogurt, simply pour some condensed milk into the warm quinoa and stir through. Or, for an exotic twist, add a few drops of rose or orange blossom water to your fruit compote.

Serves 2

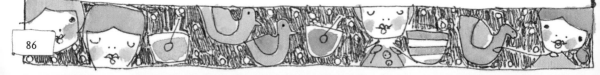

Camille's Saucepan Ginger tea for Upset tummies & Immunity

Oh no! I'm sorry to hear that you are unwell! My old friend's grandmother would always prepare this ginger tea for her; it's great for upset tummies and immunity.
Get Well soon,
Love Camille
x

CHOP ABOUT FOUR SLICES OF FRESH GINGER AND BOIL THEM IN A POT OF WATER. LEAVE IT TO REDUCE TO ABOUT HALF (ABOUT 30 MINUTES) POUR INTO YOUR FAVOURITE CUP OR MUG, AND ADD A LITTLE HONEY AND LEMON AS DESIRED. ENJOY!

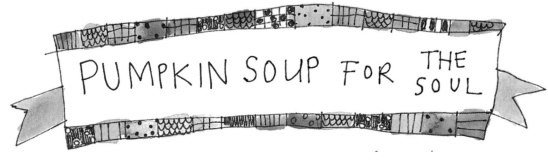

PUMPKIN SOUP FOR THE SOUL

This marvellous get-well concoction is sure to warm, nourish and comfort you. It is easy to prepare, and a treat to eat.

GINGER AND TURMERIC ARE WONDERFULLY HEALING SPICES that can balance and uplift us in daily life. Pepper helps to activate turmeric's medicinal properties, and works like a dream here, combined with grounding root vegetables and the sweetness of 'Kumera', or sweet potato. Roasting your vegetables enhances their flavour, sweetness and depth.

Enjoy ♥

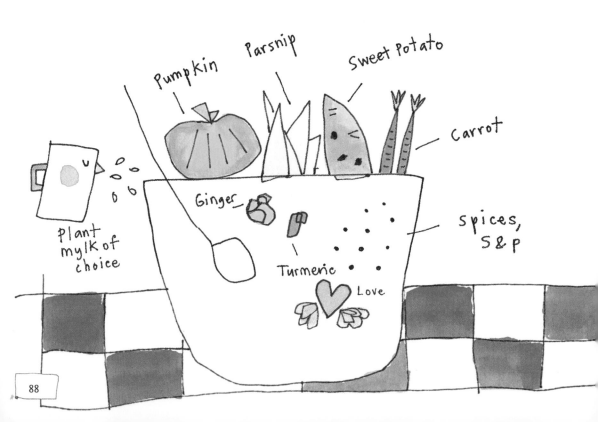

Pumpkin

Parsnip

Sweet Potato

Carrot

Ginger

spices, S & P

Plant mylk of choice

Turmeric

Love

large pumpkin
2 medium sweet potatoes
2 large carrots, diced
2 medium parsnips
3 tablespoons coconut oil
½ teaspoon cinnamon, ground
½ teaspoon coriander, ground
1 teaspoon cumin, ground
1 teaspoon turmeric, ground

1 tablespoon fresh ginger, grated
2 tablespoons almond butter
½ cup plant mylk (such as almond or
   coconut)

To serve

leafy greens, fresh herbs, pumpkin seeds,
   wholegrain bread, dollops of coconut
   yogurt

Preheat oven to 200°C (400°F).

Peel and chop the pumpkin, sweet
potatoes, carrots and parsnips into
chunks. In a large mixing bowl toss the
vegetables lightly in coconut oil, ground
spices and season with salt and pepper to
taste.

Arrange evenly on baking trays. Bake for
30 minutes, or until lightly golden and soft
when pressed with a fork.

Place the roasted vegetables into a large
saucepan and add filtered water until just
covered. Add the ginger, almond butter
and plant mylk of choice. Heat until

simmering gently then cook for about
ten minutes, stirring well to combine and
mashing the roasted vegetables gently
together.

For a chunky soup serve as is, alternatively
for a smoother, thinner consistency, add a
little more plant mylk and blend the soup
before serving.

Top with fresh leafy greens and herbs,
pumpkin seeds. Serve with a side of
toasted wholegrain bread if desired,
and a dollop of coconut yogurt if feeling
decadent!

Serves 4–6

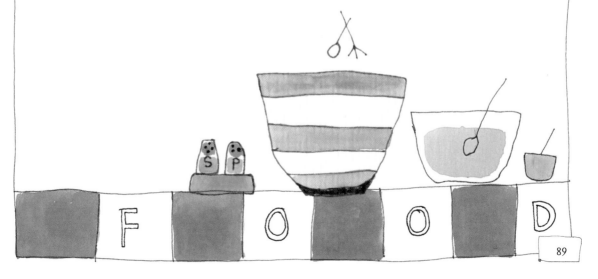

LEAFY GREEN SALAD WITH CARAMELISED HAZELNUTS AND MORE ♥

For a nutritious, calming and colour rich salad, try this exciting combination! You'll see cherries, hazelnuts, potatoes and dark leafy greens from the 'sleepy Supermarket Trolley', ingredients to encourage restfulness. This makes a lovely light dinner to welcome glorious sleep.

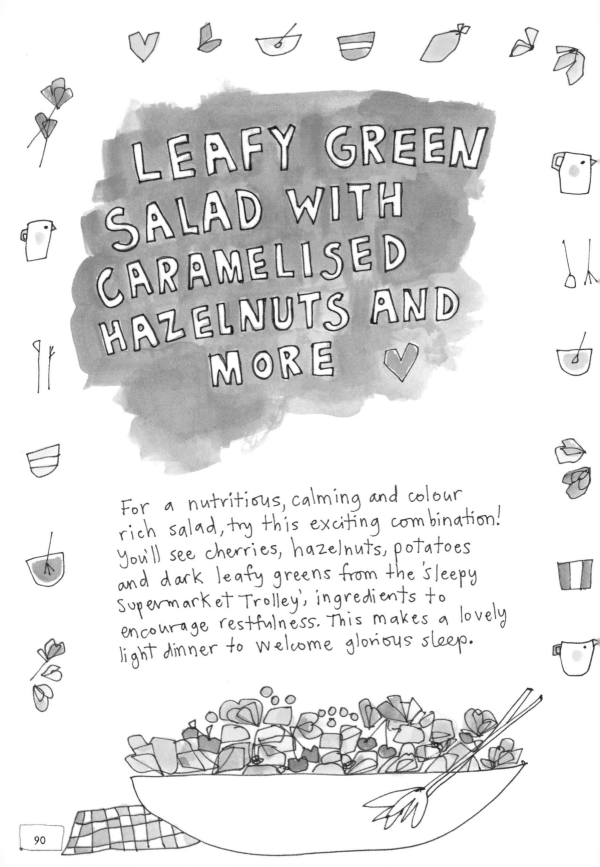

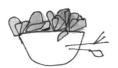

2 medium sweet potatoes, chopped into chunky rounds

1–2 tablespoons coconut oil

2 handfuls of hazelnuts

1½ tablespoons tamari (wheat free soy sauce)

1½ tablespoons pure maple syrup

3 generous handfuls of mixed baby lettuce leaves

1 generous handful of baby kale leaves

a handful of coriander leaves (optional)

a handful of halved cherry tomatoes

a handful of baby radishes, sliced

1 cucumber, sliced into rounds

1 avocado, peeled and sliced

To serve

2 tablespoons tahini

2 tablespoons lemon juice

1 teaspoon lemon zest

1 heaped teaspoon pure wholegrain mustard

⅓ cup of warm filtered water

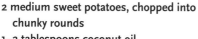

Preheat oven to 200°C (400°F) degrees.

Rub the sweet potato pieces in coconut oil and season to taste with salt and pepper. Bake for about 25–30 minutes, turning once after 15 minutes. They will be done when they are golden and crispy on the outside, soft and chewy inside.

Meanwhile, place a frypan over a low heat and toss in the hazelnuts. Once warm, add the tamari and pure maple syrup and stir to combine. Allow the hazelnuts to caramelise but not burn! Keep a close eye on them. Once they're sticky and delicious, remove them from the pan and set aside on a plate. Separate them gently with a fork.

Wash and drain the leafy greens and place in a mixing bowl with the coriander, radishes, tomatoes and cucumber. Toss well to combine.

Place all the dressing ingredients in a little jug and whisk well. Season to taste with salt and pepper, and add extra warm water until your desired pouring consistency is achieved.

Arrange the salad on your favourite serving plates. Once the sweet potatoes are ready, arrange them on top with avocado slices and a sprinkling of caramelised hazelnuts. Drizzle liberally with dressing to finish. Sit back, relax and enjoy!

Serves 2–4

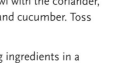

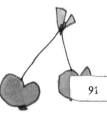

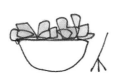

THE 'COMFORT ME!' CRUMBLE

When on the hunt for something warm, delicious and nurturing, you can't go past a good crumble. This wonderful recipe for sour cherry and apple crumble is decadently accompanied by coconut yogurt.

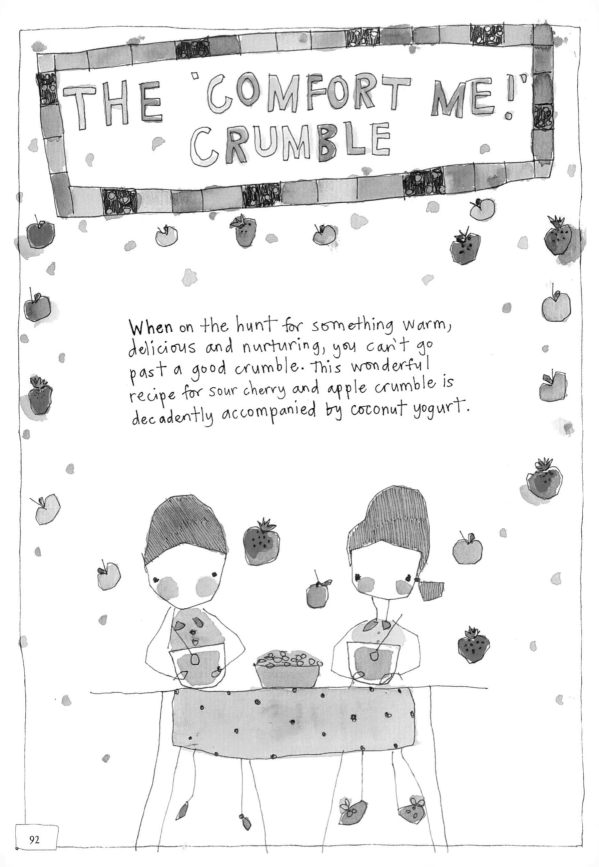

350 g (12 oz) organic sour cherries
8 small (or 4 large) green apples, peeled,
    cored and thinly sliced
2 teaspoons of pure vanilla essence

CRUMBLE TOPPING
90 g (3 oz) butter, melted
½ cup almonds, roughly chopped
½ cup macadamia nuts, roughly chopped

⅓ cup almond meal
½ cup shredded coconut
⅓ teaspoon cinnamon
1 little pinch of salt
2 tablespoons coconut oil, melted
3½ tablespoons pure maple syrup
1–2 teaspoons grated lemon zest
1 tablespoon of lemon juice

Combine the sour cherries, apples and vanilla in a saucepan. Add filtered water to just cover. Bring to the boil and reduce to a gentle simmer for about half an hour, stirring occasionally until a syrupy, compote like consistency is achieved.

Preheat oven to 180°C (350°F).

Add all the topping ingredients to a mixing bowl and stir well to combine.

When the compote is cooked, pour it into a ceramic baking dish (or individual ramekins if desired, this recipe fills four of mine) and sprinkle the topping evenly across the top.

Bake for 15 minutes, or until lightly golden on top.

Serve with coconut yogurt, love, and a pot of tea.

Serves 4–6

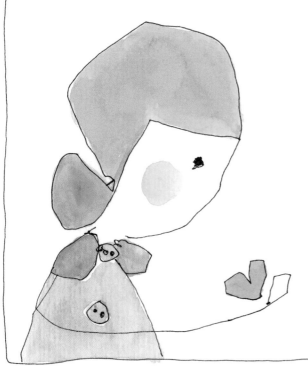

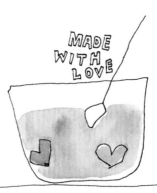

MADE
WITH
LOVE

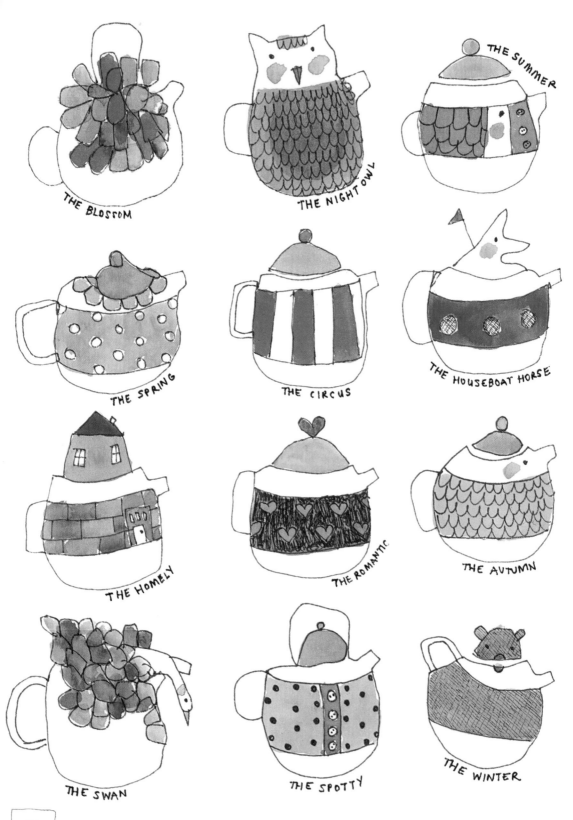

THE BLOSSOM

THE NIGHT OWL

THE SUMMER

THE SPRING

THE CIRCUS

THE HOUSEBOAT HORSE

THE HOMELY

THE ROMANTIC

THE AUTUMN

THE SWAN

THE SPOTTY

THE WINTER

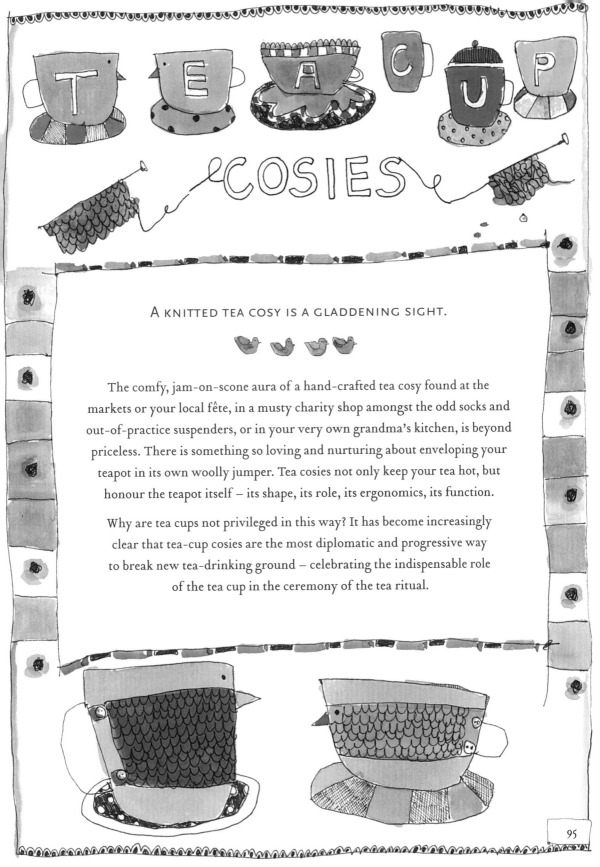

TEA CUP COSIES

A KNITTED TEA COSY IS A GLADDENING SIGHT.

The comfy, jam-on-scone aura of a hand-crafted tea cosy found at the markets or your local fête, in a musty charity shop amongst the odd socks and out-of-practice suspenders, or in your very own grandma's kitchen, is beyond priceless. There is something so loving and nurturing about enveloping your teapot in its own woolly jumper. Tea cosies not only keep your tea hot, but honour the teapot itself – its shape, its role, its ergonomics, its function.

Why are tea cups not privileged in this way? It has become increasingly clear that tea-cup cosies are the most diplomatic and progressive way to break new tea-drinking ground – celebrating the indispensable role of the tea cup in the ceremony of the tea ritual.

HOW TO MAKE YOUR OWN TEA CUP COSY:

You will need:

3mm needles
a ball of 4 ply wool
(eg: Zarina Chine Extra Fine)
3 small (10mm) buttons.

Cast on 45 stitches and work 4 rows in K1, P1 rib.

5th row (right side): Purl.

6th row: Knit, increasing 1 stitch at each end of row.

Continue in stocking stitch (1 row purl, 1 row knit), increasing 1 stitch at each end of every 4th row (10th, 14th, 18th, 22nd, 26th, 30th, 34th and 38th rows).

You should have 63 stitches!

KNIT: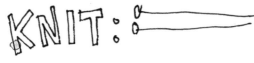

ME

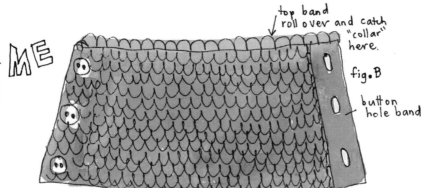

top band
roll over and catch "collar" here.

fig. B

button hole band

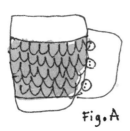

Fig. A

TOP BAND

39th row (right side): Knit.

40th row: Purl.

Continue in stocking stitch, without shaping, for a further 15 rows.

Next row: Cast off in K1, P1 rib.

BUTTONHOLE BAND

Cast on 5 stitches, and work 2 rows in K1, Pl rib.

3rd row (buttonhole row): K1, P1, cast off 2 stitches, K1.

4th row: K1, cast on two stitches, K1, P1.

Continue working in rib, making a buttonhole, as above, in the 21st and 22nd rows, and the 39th and 40th rows.

Knit 2 more rows in K1, P1 rib.

Next row: Cast off in K1, P1 rib.

MAKING UP

Using a needle and thread (ideally a blunt 'wool' needle and a length of wool) and with right side facing, attach buttonhole band to the left side of your cosy (see diagram on previous page).

The top band should naturally roll down to form a 'collar' – using a needle and thread, secure the rolled collar at each side edge.

Sew three small buttons to the right side of the cosy to line up with the buttonholes, and voilà, it's now ready to snuggle up to your cup – and warm your favourite brew!

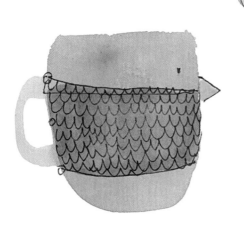

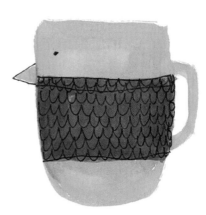

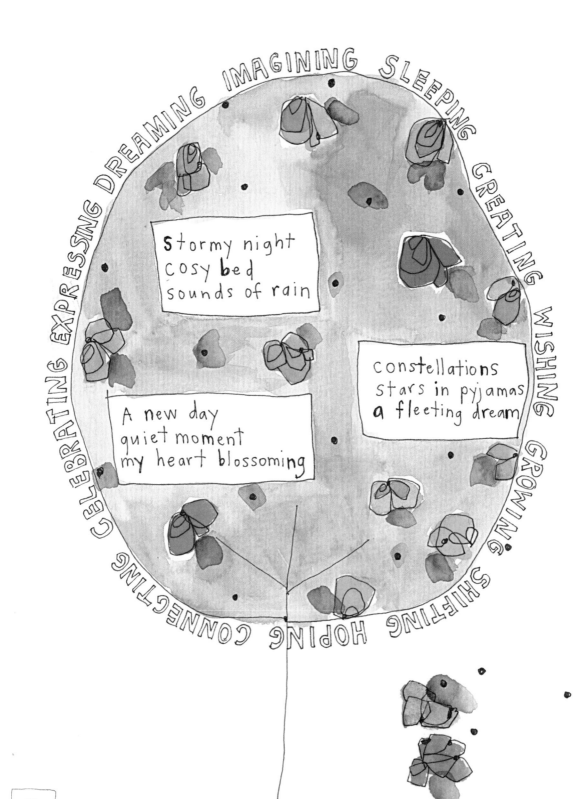

Stormy night
cosy bed
sounds of rain

constellations
stars in pyjamas
a fleeting dream

A new day
quiet moment
my heart blossoming

IMAGINING SLEEPING CREATING WISHING GROWING SHIFTING HOPING CONNECTING CELEBRATING EXPRESSING DREAMING

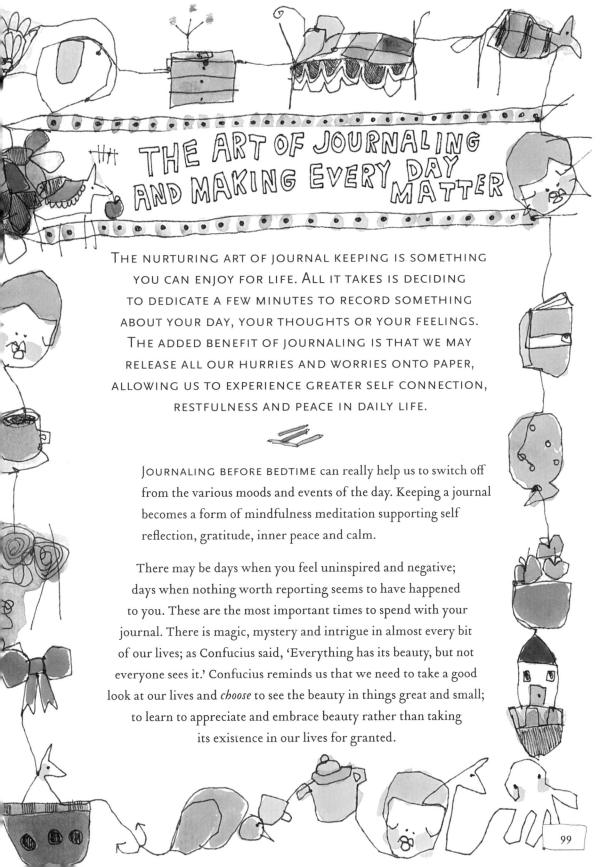

THE ART OF JOURNALING AND MAKING EVERY DAY MATTER

THE NURTURING ART OF JOURNAL KEEPING IS SOMETHING YOU CAN ENJOY FOR LIFE. ALL IT TAKES IS DECIDING TO DEDICATE A FEW MINUTES TO RECORD SOMETHING ABOUT YOUR DAY, YOUR THOUGHTS OR YOUR FEELINGS. THE ADDED BENEFIT OF JOURNALING IS THAT WE MAY RELEASE ALL OUR HURRIES AND WORRIES ONTO PAPER, ALLOWING US TO EXPERIENCE GREATER SELF CONNECTION, RESTFULNESS AND PEACE IN DAILY LIFE.

JOURNALING BEFORE BEDTIME can really help us to switch off from the various moods and events of the day. Keeping a journal becomes a form of mindfulness meditation supporting self reflection, gratitude, inner peace and calm.

There may be days when you feel uninspired and negative; days when nothing worth reporting seems to have happened to you. These are the most important times to spend with your journal. There is magic, mystery and intrigue in almost every bit of our lives; as Confucius said, 'Everything has its beauty, but not everyone sees it.' Confucius reminds us that we need to take a good look at our lives and *choose* to see the beauty in things great and small; to learn to appreciate and embrace beauty rather than taking its existence in our lives for granted.

LOOK AT YOUR TEA CUP. Every tea cup has a different shape and feeling. Does it have little cracks? Tea stains? What does it feel like to hold? Now take a pencil, close your eyes and draw it. It doesn't matter whether your drawing looks like a tea cup or not; the stranger the better. Now grab colours, ones that match your state of mind. Write a few words around your cup – describe your mood. This alone is a wonderful start.

DRAW ANYTHING you see: objects in your bedroom, the shape of a window, the sleeping pet at the end of your bed. Closing your eyes and drawing allows you to *feel* objects and frees you from expecting a perfect end result. Study the shapes and textures of the world around you: sounds, words, overheard conversations, beeps of machines, and the rhythms of footsteps. Being aware of and appreciating the beauty of small things will make your days richer, your imagination wilder and your heart more joyful.

YOUR JOURNAL IS also a wonderful place to record your dreams. Writing them down encourages you to remember them, and even promotes dreaming. The more attention you pay to your dreams the more messages from your subconscious you will receive. These are important and can guide you on your life's path. Keeping tickets, snippets of letters, postcards, pieces of fabric, buttons or photographs will also become important, as these tactile things hold their own memories and add texture and dimension to your craft and your life.

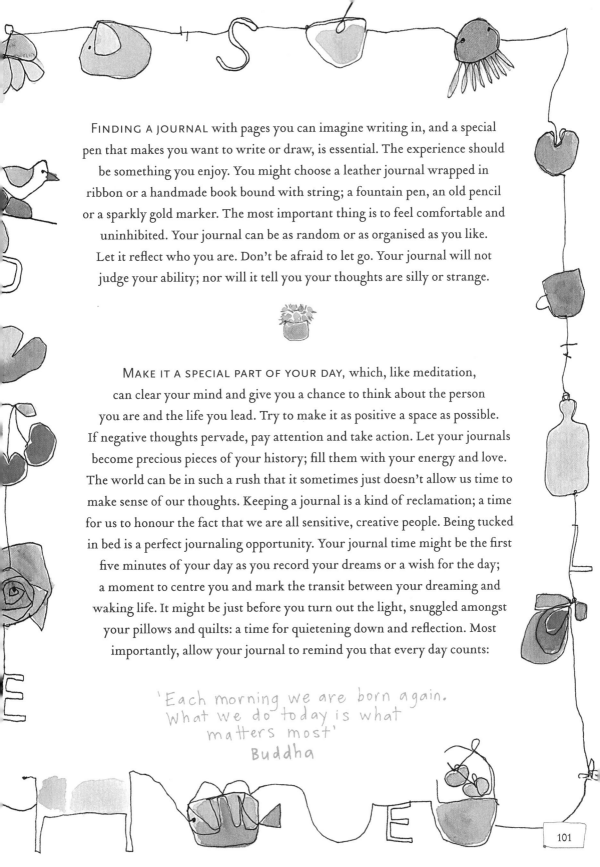

FINDING A JOURNAL with pages you can imagine writing in, and a special pen that makes you want to write or draw, is essential. The experience should be something you enjoy. You might choose a leather journal wrapped in ribbon or a handmade book bound with string; a fountain pen, an old pencil or a sparkly gold marker. The most important thing is to feel comfortable and uninhibited. Your journal can be as random or as organised as you like. Let it reflect who you are. Don't be afraid to let go. Your journal will not judge your ability; nor will it tell you your thoughts are silly or strange.

MAKE IT A SPECIAL PART OF YOUR DAY, which, like meditation, can clear your mind and give you a chance to think about the person you are and the life you lead. Try to make it as positive a space as possible. If negative thoughts pervade, pay attention and take action. Let your journals become precious pieces of your history; fill them with your energy and love. The world can be in such a rush that it sometimes just doesn't allow us time to make sense of our thoughts. Keeping a journal is a kind of reclamation; a time for us to honour the fact that we are all sensitive, creative people. Being tucked in bed is a perfect journaling opportunity. Your journal time might be the first five minutes of your day as you record your dreams or a wish for the day; a moment to centre you and mark the transit between your dreaming and waking life. It might be just before you turn out the light, snuggled amongst your pillows and quilts: a time for quietening down and reflection. Most importantly, allow your journal to remind you that every day counts:

'Each morning we are born again.
What we do today is what
matters most'
Buddha

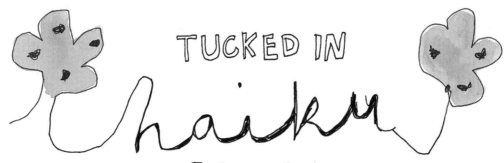

TUCKED IN

haiku

POETRY

SELF EXPRESSION IS ESSENTIAL TO A FUN AND RELAXING LIFE IN WHICH REST AND PLAY ARE BEAUTIFULLY BALANCED. PUTTING PEN TO PAPER HAS ITS OWN HEALING POWER, AND TIME TUCKED IN BED IS THE PERFECT TIME TO CONNECT WITH YOUR INNER POET!

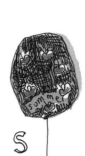

Haiku, originating in Japan, refers to a form of poetry composed traditionally of seventeen syllables arranged into three lines. Describing haiku in Western terms, however, involves some degree of syncretism. Syllables are Western measures of sound units; the actual Japanese term to measure is the *mora*, which is not quite the same thing as a syllable, but probably its closest equivalent. The words and units inevitably change when haiku is translated into English from Japanese, too. The traditional rhythm for the haiku arrangement was five, seven, five *moras* (otherwise known as simply *on*). We may take for example, 'Old Pond' by Bashō, one of the best known of Japanese haiku poets:

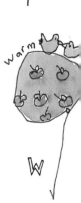

古池や 蛙飛込む 水の音

This divides into:

fu-ru-i-ke ya (5)
ka-wa-zu to-bi-ko-mu (7)
mi-zu no o-to (5)

Translated

old pond...
a frog leaps in
water's sound

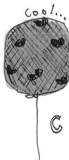

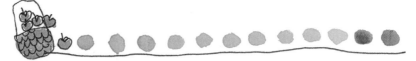

BASHŌ'S PROLIFIC EXPRESSION through haiku closely links to his Zen Buddhism. His poetry is infused with Buddhist ideas and teachings which recognise and succinctly capture the essence of being. Traditional haiku themes are usually inspired by nature and the place of humans within the wider world. A particular emphasis was often placed on the life of the seasons and the flow of time.

With the passing of the years and the journey of haiku poetry through many lands, its form has become more flexible and its formal boundaries blurred. It has retained, however, its concise character, and is still usually composed of seventeen syllables or fewer altogether, arranged into three lines.

WITH A FOCUS ON the openness and simplicity of haiku we can explore our inner poet. With no rules about rhyming words, complex themes or making perfect sense, writing our own variations of haiku is a wonderful way to begin noticing, celebrating and documenting the marvellous, unusual, perhaps seemingly banal things that we see and feel. The beauty of haiku is often in the capturing of a moment in its pure and unembellished form. Let yourself see the world through curious, grateful eyes, and allow a new sense of richness to permeate your days.

I hope the ease of Haiku might inspire you to take pen to paper whilst tucked in, perhaps even revealing a wonderful, untapped talent just waiting to be explored! You might like to visit the poem tree on page 98 for a little inspiration.

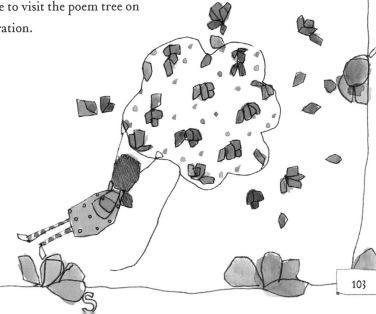

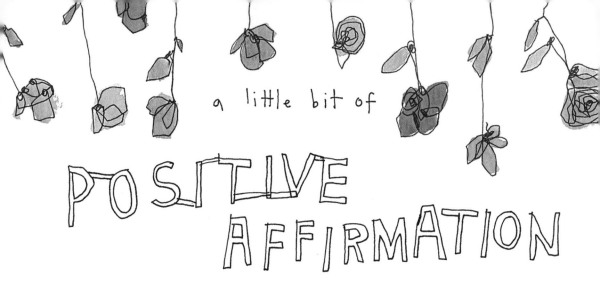

a little bit of POSITIVE AFFIRMATION

ON THE ROLLERCOASTER OF LIFE WE EXPERIENCE WONDERFUL HIGHS —
LOVE, CREATIVITY, MOTIVATION AND FEELINGS OF CONNECTEDNESS;
WE SMILE, WE LAUGH, WE FEEL BRAVE AND IN CONTROL.

These moments cannot be recognised and appreciated for what they are without
the contrasting emotions of sadness and pain which are also natural in the human
experience. You might be tucked in feeling sad, unwell, exhausted or uninspired.
On these darker, harder days it is sometimes hard to rustle up the warm, positive
feelings we need to affirm and comfort us. We are not alone in these times.
Simply thinking of life as a shared experience, of each individual as a unique
being with his or her own struggles and ups and downs, can bring a sense
of perspective and harmony back to our hearts.

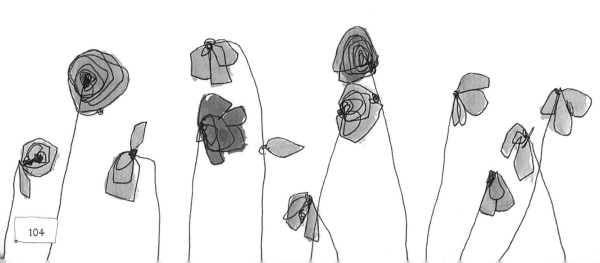

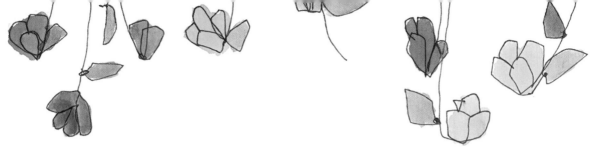

Reminders that we are okay can be sought from the outside world;
from friends and family whose encouragement and support is so essential
to our feelings of strength and belonging. However, the most important person
to look to is yourself; to realise the full potential of your spirit and inner strength,
and to trust in yourself to carry you on your path through life. Being sensitive
to and honest about your emotions is a wonderful start.

ACKNOWLEDGING WHEN YOU need to rest, to take a little bit of time out, is not always
an easy thing in this busy world where machines and people move so fast. Televisions,
computers, mobile phones, cars, pagers and clocks all bombard us with pictures and
sounds, polluting our potential quiet times with stressful disruptions. Tucking in
and simply enjoying the feeling, quietly appreciating the cosiness of bed, a wonderful
book or a good cup of tea, is okay, and is in fact completely necessary. We must allow
ourselves to feel tired and to fully appreciate the replenishing, healing nature of sleep
and rest. Listening to our bodies is the least we can do; they are the only ones that
we have and they deserve our love and attention.

These little affirmation cards (on pages 106–107) are for you, particularly on those
harder days when you might need to remind yourself that you have what it takes
to navigate the wild and woolly oceans of life. You are strong enough, you are patient
enough; you are your best self. Focus on these positive affirmations and watch the way
your spirit will naturally attract good things into your life. The recipe is simple but
foolproof – our lives are gifts to be experienced fully in all their diversity and richness.

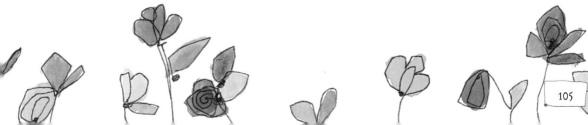

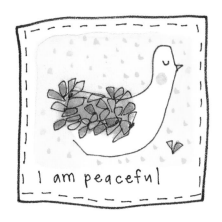

I am peaceful

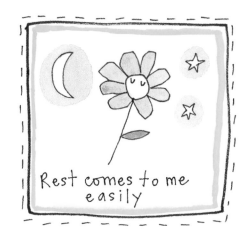

Rest comes to me easily

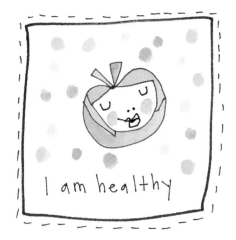

I am healthy

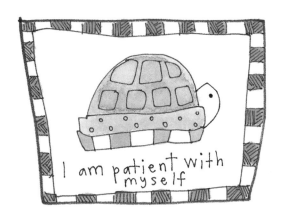

I am patient with myself

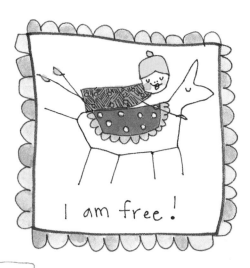

I am free!

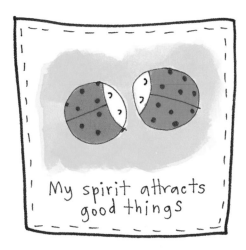

My spirit attracts good things

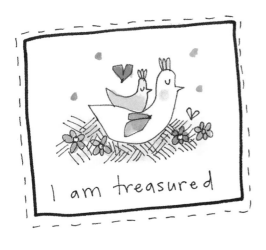

I am treasured

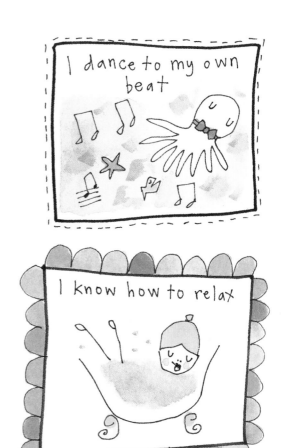

I dance to my own beat

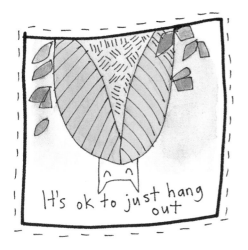

It's ok to just hang out

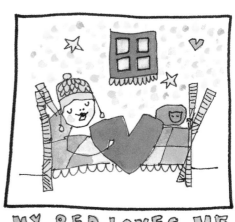

I know how to relax

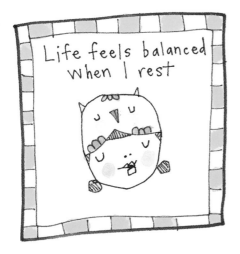

Life feels balanced when I rest

MY BED LOVES ME

Little Meditations
ENJOYING LIFE'S QUIET MOMENTS

THE WONDERS OF MEDITATION CAN
BE ENJOYED IN MANY FORMS. ANY RELAXING PRACTICE OF
SELF CARE WILL CONTRIBUTE PROFOUNDLY TO CULTIVATING
RESTFULNESS IN DAILY LIFE.

While formal types of meditation can be taught and learnt, other ways of quietening your mind which don't involve much discipline at all can be tucked easily into your day. Simply lighting a candle and taking a moment to watch the flame, or paying attention to the sensation of your breath as it goes in and out of your mouth and nose, are great places to start. Your meditation time might be a quiet cup of tea at the end of your day, allowing yourself a moment to gather your thoughts and reflect in peace. Looking out over the ocean, the mountains, or up into the stars might be your way of meditating; allowing you to reconnect with the essence of your spirit and your being.

These quiet moments are not only essential counterpoints in our busy lives; they ground us and remind us to reaffirm our priorities. They relax us, and contribute to our enjoyment of rest.

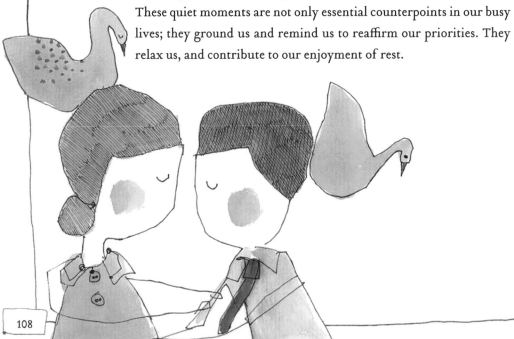

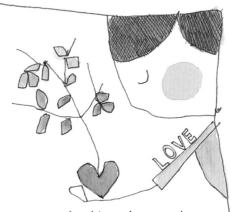

T HE THINGS THAT WE SEE EVERY DAY, the things that constitute our own image slide show, stimulate our emotions. They might be particular views, faces of friends, family and colleagues, even colours. We can actively seek to fill our lives with beautiful pictures, warm colours and friendly faces. We can choose to see the beauty and the good in our days, even when they may seem less than perfect. By simply appreciating the magnificence in small things, you will feel a new sense of gratitude to sustain and inspire you. As an added bonus, mindful living usually leads to our unique needs being met, making way for greater rest and relaxation in daily life. Take care in creating uplifting environments in your home and workplace; embrace colours, textures and sounds that make you feel good. Make your day-to-day life feel special: have a favourite tea cup, bring in some fresh flowers, make your bed and take time to set the table. Do all that you do with a sense of awareness, and you will experience the feelings of peace and balance that you seek. By approaching your life with open eyes and awareness you will find that almost everything you do can become a meditative experience.

The following images and meditations are for you to simply sink into. The words and images focus on positive thinking and encourage you to spend a quiet moment with yourself. Your days can be tiresome and dreary, or they can be abundant – you have the opportunity to choose. Your life is what you make it.

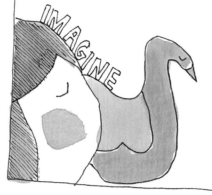

Live the life you dream of.

and today ?..
. . . .

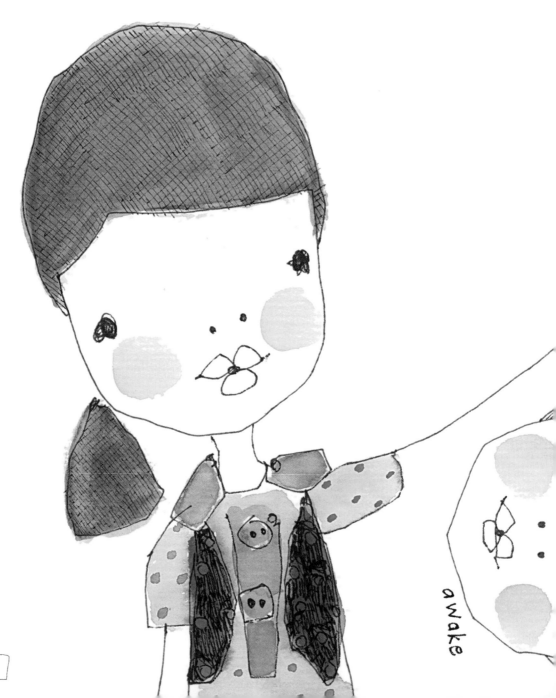

awake

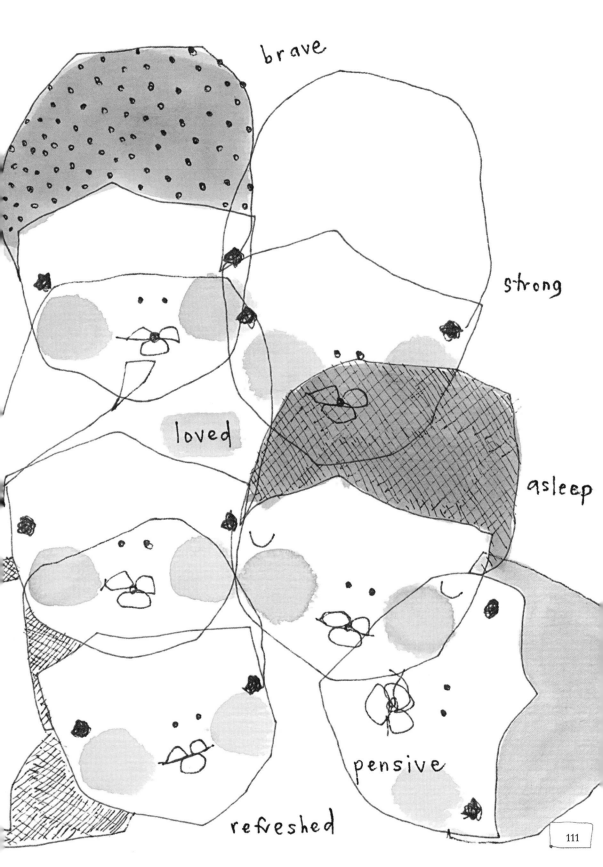

brave

strong

loved

asleep

refreshed

pensive

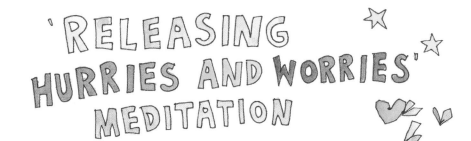

'RELEASING HURRIES AND WORRIES' MEDITATION

A relaxing meditation to support restfulness.

As I lie here and gently close my eyes, I take a moment to release my hurries and worries.

I let go of all things I need to do and all the places I need to be.

I place my hands lightly over my belly and feel it rise and fall.

I simply breathe deeply now, in and out.

In this moment I let go of myself.

I let go of any thoughts I have about myself, good, bad or in between.

I let myself breathe peacefully.

Breathing slowly on; in and out.

I feel each part of my body now, from my head to my toes.

When I lie here softly, I let myself feel whole and complete.

As a I breathe deeply I feel lighter. Rest comes easily to me.

I let myself feel restful, and relax into blissful sleep.

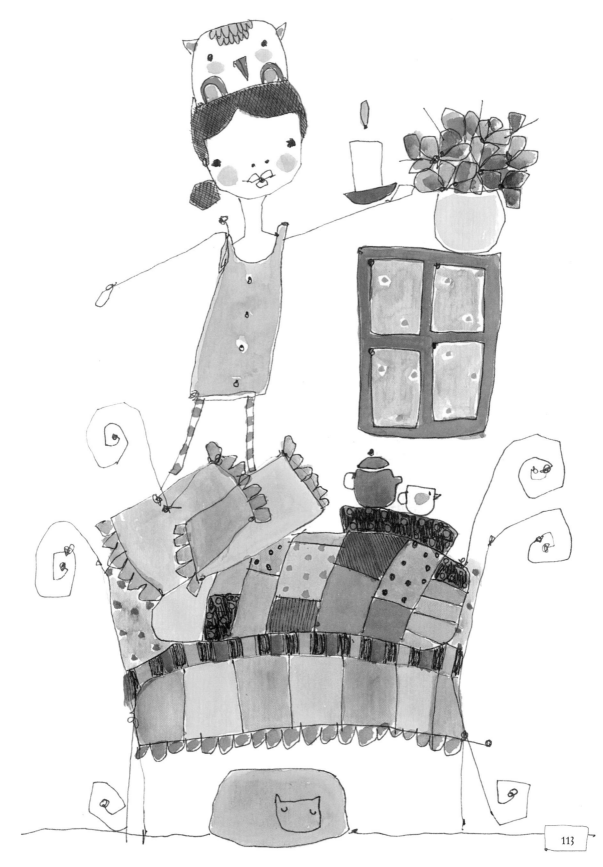

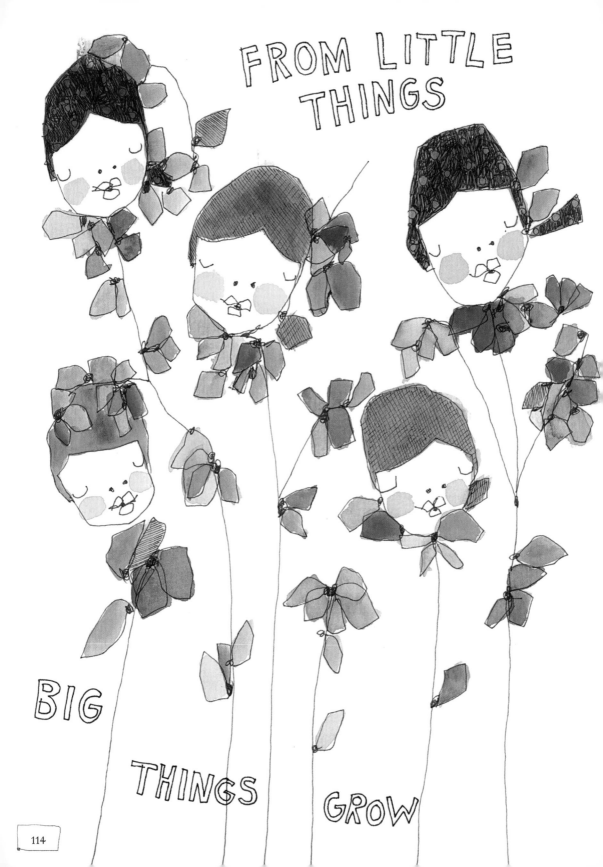

FROM LITTLE THINGS

BIG THINGS GROW

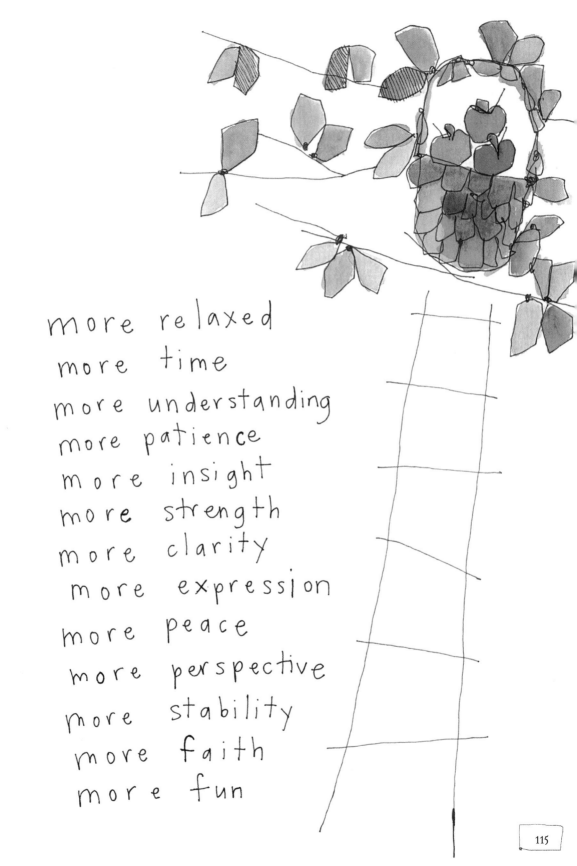

more relaxed
more time
more understanding
more patience
more insight
more strength
more clarity
more expression
more peace
more perspective
more stability
more faith
more fun

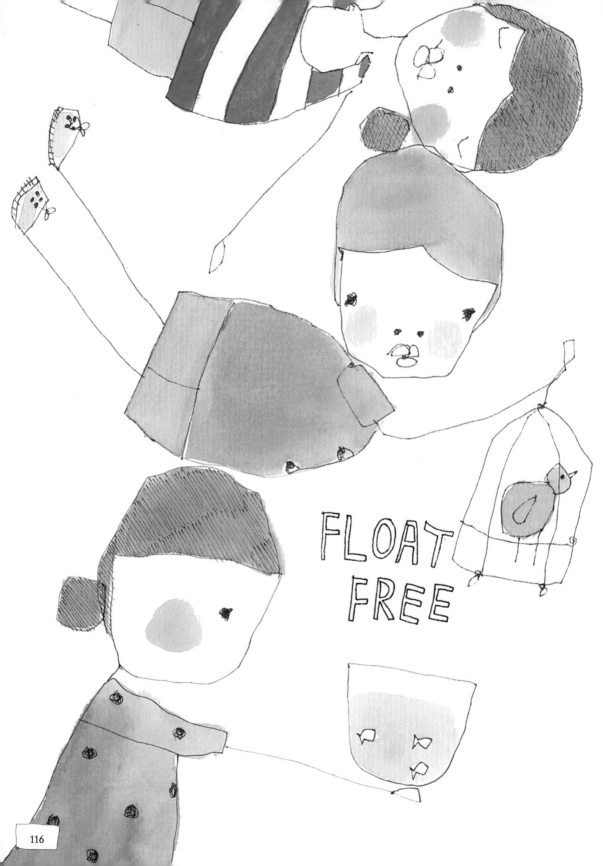

FLOAT
FREE

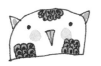

'READY FOR DREAMY ADVENTURES' MEDITATION ☆ ☆

A meditation to sink into a deliciously dreamy state and relish the joy and whimsy of sleep.

TONIGHT AS I PREPARE FOR SLEEP, I let myself feel ready for the adventures that await me in my dreams. I ask myself, 'Where would you like to go tonight?'

Would I like to potter through a rainforest or climb a mountain? Would I like to travel to a tropical paradise or fly through the stars?

As I breathe gently now, in and out, I let my imagination float freely.

My dreams await me every night, ready to whisk me away on infinite adventures.

I take a moment now to think about and feel thankful for the magic of my dreams.

As I relax, I float gently into the colours, the sights and the sounds of a new adventure.

As I relax even more deeply, I drift gently off to sleep ...

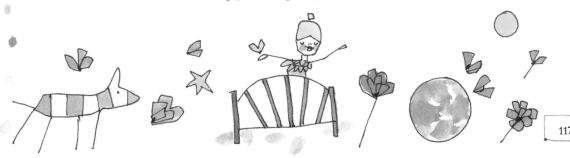

'MY BED LOVES ME' MEDITATION ♥

A meditation to acknowledge your bed's unconditional love.

As I TUCK IN TONIGHT, I take a moment to notice that my bed loves me.

My bed is always here for me, forever supporting me to rest and relax.

My bed always holds me up and nestles me in.

On good days and bad days, my bed waits patiently for me.

My bed never judges me, it loves me to snuggle up and feel peaceful.

My bed is always cosy. I feel safe and sound when I come to bed.

At last the hurries, worries and stresses of my day can melt into my dreams.

With this little prayer, I thank my bed for loving me, and let myself drift softly into sleep.

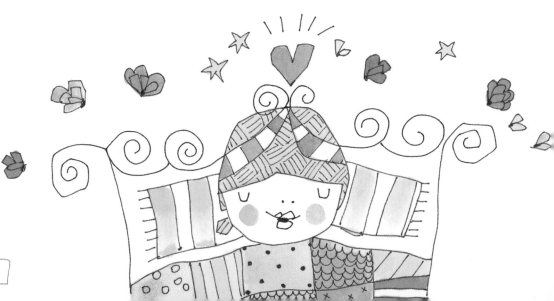

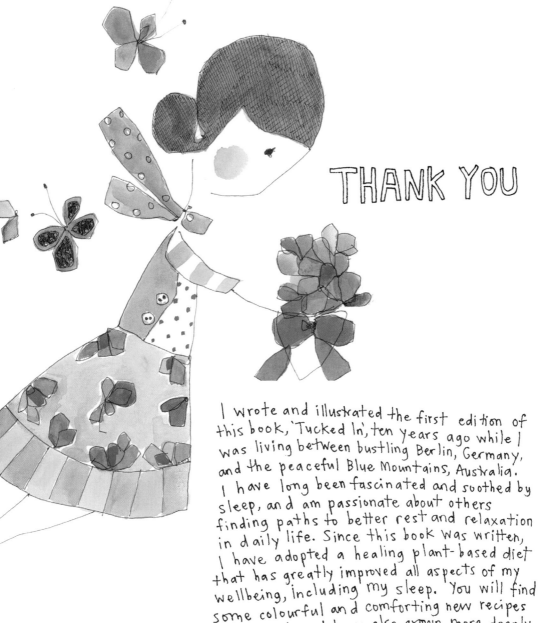

THANK YOU

I wrote and illustrated the first edition of this book, 'Tucked In', ten years ago while I was living between bustling Berlin, Germany, and the peaceful Blue Mountains, Australia. I have long been fascinated and soothed by sleep, and am passionate about others finding paths to better rest and relaxation in daily life. Since this book was written, I have adopted a healing plant-based diet that has greatly improved all aspects of my wellbeing, including my sleep. You will find some colourful and comforting new recipes to try within. I have also grown more deeply passionate about mindfulness and included extra meditations into this edition for your enjoyment. I thank Pam Brewster and the team at Hardie Grant for releasing this book again, and allowing me to breathe new life into it. I thank all my readers past, present and future for enjoying my books.

I wish you sweet dreams, and send you my love,

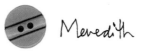 Meredith

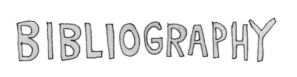

BIBLIOGRAPHY

Ten Thousand Dreams Interpreted by
Gustavus Hindman Miller, Elements,
Shaftsbury, England, 1996

Basho - The Complete Haiku by Matsuo
Basho, translated by Jane Reichhold,
Kondansha International, Tokyo, 2008

Celtic Lullabies, Various artists. Compiled
by Jill Rogoff (CD) 1994. Ellipsis Arts

Chuang - Tsu: Basic Writings of Zuangzi,
translated by Burton Watson, Columbia
University Press, New York 1964

The Planet Sleeps, Various artists. Compiled
by David Field (CD) 1997. Sony

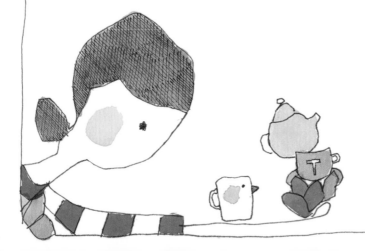

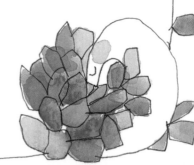

Published in 2018 by Hardie Grant
an imprint of Hardie Grant Publishing

Hardie Grant Books (Melbourne)
Building 1, 658 Church Street
Richmond VIC 3121

Hardie Grant London
5th & 6th Floors
52-54 Southwark Street
London SE1 1UN

hardiegrantbooks.com

A cataloguing-in-Publication entry is available from
the catalogue of the National Library of Australia
www.nla.gov.au

Your Bed Loves You
ISBN 978 1 74379 421 0

Publisher: Pam Brewster
Designer: Arielle Gamble
Production Manager: Todd Rechner

Colour reproduction by Splitting Image Colour studio

Printed in China by 1010 Printing International Limited

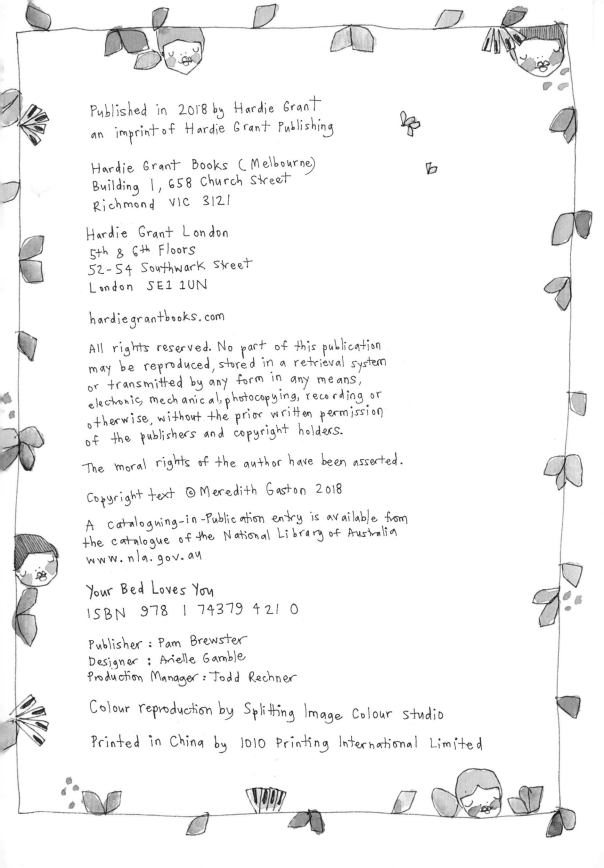

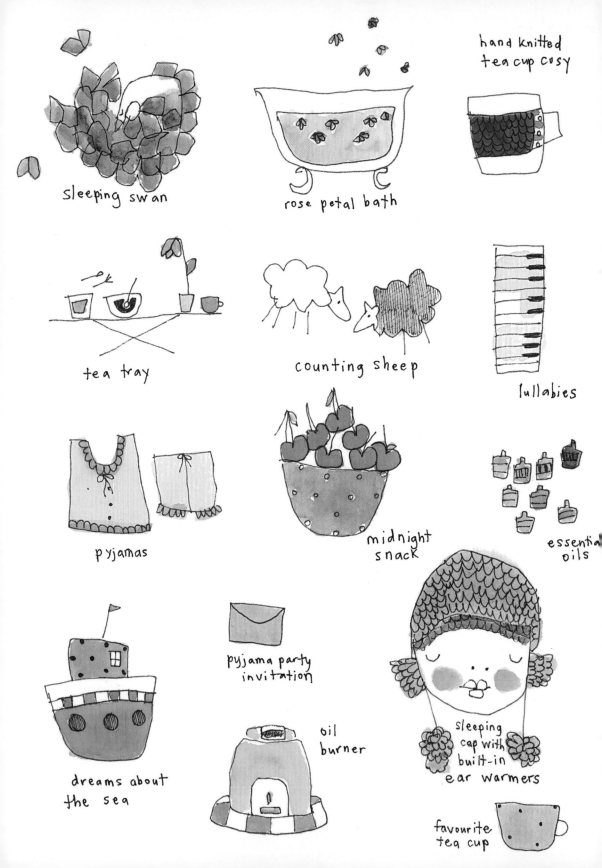

sleeping swan

rose petal bath

hand knitted tea cup cosy

tea tray

counting sheep

lullabies

pyjamas

midnight snack

essential oils

dreams about the sea

pyjama party invitation

oil burner

sleeping cap with built-in ear warmers

favourite tea cup